THE WESTMINSTER SERIES

General Editor: W. A. J. FARNDALE

VOLUME 8

THE PRINCIPLES AND PRACTICE OF HEALTH VISITING

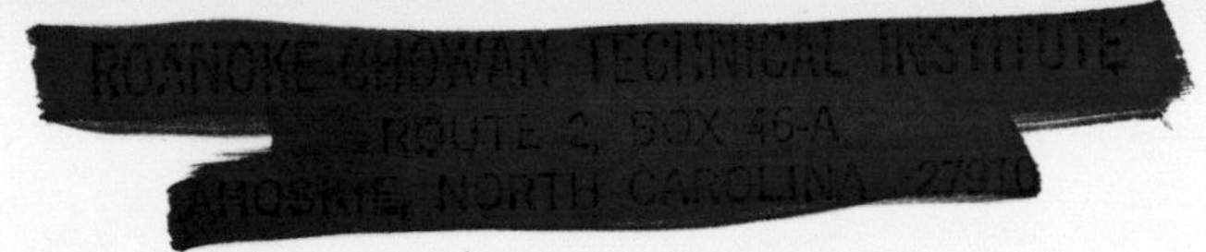

THE PRINCIPLES AND PRACTICE OF HEALTH VISITING

by

ROSEMARY HALE
S.R.N., S.C.M., H.V. Cert., Dip. Soc. Sc. (Lond.)., F.R.S.H
Late Lecturer and Principal Health Visitor Tutor, University of Surrey

MARION K. LOVELAND
S.R.N., S.C.M., D.N. (Lond.)., Q.N., H.V.Cert.
Lecturer, Health Visitor Course, University of Surrey

GRACE M. OWEN
S.R.N., S.C.M., Q.N., H.V. Tutor's Cert., F.R.S.H.
Lecturer, Health Visitor Course, University of Surrey

With an introduction by

IAN A. G. MACQUEEN
O.B.E., M.A., M.D., D.P.H., F.R.S.H.
Medical Officer of Health, Principal School Medical Officer, Port Medical Officer and Director of Welfare, City of Aberdeen

PERGAMON PRESS
OXFORD · LONDON · EDINBURGH · NEW YORK
TORONTO · SYDNEY · PARIS · BRAUNSCHWEIG

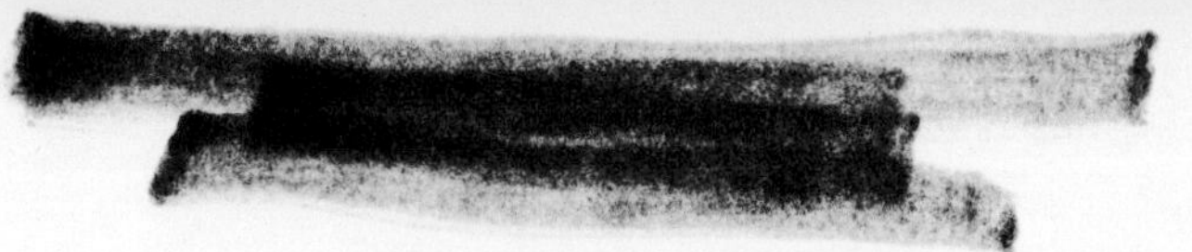

Pergamon Press Ltd., Headington Hill Hall, Oxford
4 & 5 Fitzroy Square, London W.1
Pergamon Press (Scotland) Ltd., 2 & 3 Teviot Place, Edinburgh 1
Pergamon Press Inc., 44–01 21st Street, Long Island City, New York 11101
Pergamon of Canada, Ltd., 6 Adelaide Street East, Toronto, Ontario
Pergamon Press (Aust.) Pty. Ltd., Rushcutters Bay, Sydney, N.S.W.
Pergamon Press S.A.R.L., 24 rue des Écoles, Paris 5ᵉ
Vieweg & Sohn GmbH, Burgplatz 1, Braunschweig

Copyright © 1968
Pergamon Press Ltd.

First edition 1968

15991

Library of Congress Catalog Card No. 67–31078

Filmset by The European Printing Corporation Limited, Dublin, Ireland
and printed in Great Britain by J. W. Arrowsmith Limited, Bristol

08 003575 2

To all "OLD BATS"

Contents

Rosemary Hale – a Tribute

IT IS a great sorrow to the many friends of Miss Hale that she did not see the publication of this book which contains the fruits of her accumulated experience in the teaching of health visitors. Her work in public health nursing extended over many years, twelve of them as a health visitor and a further fifteen in teaching in Battersea College of Advanced Technology, now the University of Surrey.

The contribution a teacher can make to the development of her pupils represents the synthesis of work in varied settings. Miss Hale had the opportunity of as widely varied experience as contact with a World Health Organization project in Gambia and studies of public health nursing services in Holland and the Scandinavian countries. In addition, her acceptance of the fact that work in education requires continued personal studies gave added depth to her teaching. The Health Visitor Training School at Battersea was a large one and Miss Hale, therefore, had influenced many young Health Visitors entering the service, but her contribution extended beyond this through the service she gave over the years to the professional organizations. This contact with the practising Health Visitor and colleagues in administrative positions ensured that her teaching never acquired that detachment which can so easily ensue where there is over-reliance on academic studies.

It was a matter of great interest to Miss Hale and pleasure to Council members and staff that she was one of the members of the first Council for the Training of Health Visitors and served with that body from 1962 to 1965. Here she was able to bring her long experience to the discussions which led to the formation of a new type of syllabus and a new system of examination. The culminating point in her career in teaching, however, would be the contribution that she was able to make to the institution of courses involving preparation both in nursing and in public health. She was associated with one of the first courses integrating health visiting into state registration preparation and, latterly, was closely associated with the inauguration of the Degree in Human Biology with a nursing option in the new University of Surrey. She had a full career and was able as a result to make a contribution to her profession which will not readily be forgotten by her students or her colleagues who came in contact with her. They will be glad to have this tangible record of some of her thinking in the years she gave to that profession.

June, 1967

E. E. WILKIE
Chief Professional Adviser
Council for the Training of Health Visitors

Authors' Preface

ALTHOUGH this book has been written primarily for health visitor students, we hope it will be found useful to nurse students, social workers, teachers and members of the medical profession, because we firmly believe that the surest way to good team work is a factual knowledge of the training and function of other colleagues. Particularly we hope that our book will be useful to our nursing and public health colleagues in the Commonwealth countries; also it should find a place among the careers information available to schools.

Much of the material will be individual, gleaned from our long experience in health visiting and as teachers of health visiting principles and practice. This is not a textbook because we believe that students should read recommended books on the subjects of the syllabus rather than potted extracts in a textbook.

We are grateful for the encouragement and help of our academic and secretarial colleagues in the Biological Sciences Department of the University of Surrey.

1. Introduction

Ian A. G. MacQueen

When a registered nurse with appropriate academic background and suitable personal qualities is admitted to the post-basic course for student health visitors, three main strands can perhaps be identified in the preparation that she undergoes.

From her nursing training and subsequent consolidating experience she brings certain skills, attitudes and knowledge. For instance, she has already acquired a habit of accurate observation, an ability to accept responsibility, an insight into the processes of disease, a training in physiology and human biology, a capacity for sympathy without sentimentality, a set of ethical and professional standards and a considerable knowledge of human behaviour and practical psychology. All these, sharpened and in some cases extended by her further professional education, will be constantly used in her new profession. Secondly, in her health visiting course she will study certain subjects that are common to several professions: for sociology, theoretical psychology and social medicine she will probably use the same textbooks as other students, although—like them—she will have to learn to apply her knowledge of these sciences to her particular work. Thirdly, she will have to acquire certain skills which differ from or go beyond those of most allied professions: examples are the art of obtaining relevant information with minimum questioning and without appearing to probe; the capacity to assess situations and to decide wisely whether to offer immediate help in respect of the presenting problem or to uncover underlying difficulties and provide deeper aid or to refer to another worker of different expertise or to take no action; the ability to motivate people not merely to desire better mental and physical health but to alter habits and ways of life; and the art of unobtrusively teaching individuals and groups that at first neither want to learn nor realize their ignorance. These skills and capacities involve the application of nursing, psychological and sociological knowledge, but they also involve something more—something that is the very essence of successful health visiting.

This excellent book aims to convey the rudiments of these skills and capacities. It is in no sense a substitute for textbooks on psychology, sociology, teaching methods and so on—the student will still have to read these—but is, as the title implies, an attempt to provide the groundwork of the principles and practice of health visiting.

As an introduction to what is itself an introduction let me try to answer three questions. Why do we need a new book on health visiting? Why should it be written by health visitor tutors from the University of Surrey? And for whom is it intended?

Why Another Book?

There are at least seven good reasons why a book of this nature is urgently needed.

In the first place the number of health visitors is in process of rising sharply. For some years local health authorities have been planning for large increases: published proposals by all the counties, county boroughs and London boroughs of England and Wales visualize a 46 per cent rise in the number of health visitors between 1962 and 1972; and similar increases are anticipated in Scotland and Northern Ireland. To meet these demands additional post-nursing courses are being established in various universities and colleges of technology—four new ones were approved by the Council for the Training of Health Visitors during 1965 alone—and there have also been set up several integrated courses, the majority taking students with university entrance qualifications, offering combined training in general nursing and health visiting. Despite present staff shortages—a feature of all women's professions in Britain—health visitors actually in post considerably outnumber the combined total of such other health workers as public health medical officers, local authority dental officers and public health inspectors, and vastly outstrip the combined total of all other qualified social workers employed by local authorities. From sheer numbers it follows that improvement of the emotional and social health of the people depends in large measure on health visitors, and their efficiency in turn depends largely on their professional education.

Secondly, the health visitor's functions have widened and deepened immeasurably in the last quarter of a century. Twenty-five years ago she was a nurse with some further training; she was concerned mainly with the physical well-being of mothers and babies; she dealt mostly with faulty situations that already existed; and in health departments she was regarded as little more than an auxiliary and was usually responsible to a senior medical officer. Today, while she retains a nurse's acute observation and clinical insight, she has become a family health teacher and medico-social counsellor with nursing background; she is recognized as being concerned with the health and social well-being of the entire family—with the problems of the elderly and the middle-aged no less than the young; she is quite as involved in promotion of emotional and social health (e.g. long-term reduction of maladjustment and of delinquency) as in prevention of physical illness; she works mainly by anticipatory guidance, assessing in the light of the cultural and socio-economic circumstances of a family and the attitudes and prejudice of its members the types of faulty situation likely to arise and seeking by timely and unobtrusive teaching to prevent their occurrence; she has gained full professional status; and she is responsible to her own professional head who is in turn directly answerable to the medical officer of health. Her widened duties and greatly increased responsibilities make her professional preparation all the more important.

Again, the organization of health visiting is changing. There are coming to be three big groups. (a) The biggest group so far, family health visitors with districts, coping with the emotional and social problems of families in their area from birth (or conception) to the grave; providing reassurance, support, guidance and teaching for prospective parents, parents of young children, school pupils, adolescents, adults and old people; undertaking group health education in clinics, parents' clubs and schools in their district; and consulting at discretion with general practitioners and social workers. (b) A growing group, practice-attached family health visitors, undertaking similar duties in general medical practices—a system that improves co-operation between the main clinical field-worker and the main medico-social worker and health teacher, and functions well, so long as two things are clearly appreciated: first, that in the partnership the doctor is the expert in clinical diagnosis and treatment and the health visitor is the medico-social and health teaching expert, and that neither has the skill to direct the other; and second, that, just as the family doctor is free to call in medical consultants, the family health visitor retains her full membership of the health department team and is at liberty both to consult her senior nursing officer and to call in specialized workers at need. (c) An even more rapidly growing group and perhaps the most exciting development of all, specialist health visitors with additional experience or qualifications in one aspect of health visiting. Examples of specialists are: superintendents (preferably with a higher qualification in public health nursing administration), tutors (possessing a higher qualification in teaching, educational psychology and training school administration), health education organizers (responsible for co-ordination and expansion of health teaching), group advisers (either specialized on a particular subject, such as geriatrics, or acting as general counsellors to a group of less experienced health visitors), field-work instructors (family health visitors with reduced case-loads and special responsibility for the practical education of students) and liaison health visitors (in hospitals or special clinics). Although a few generalized health visitors regret the growth of specialization—because the specialist can seldom remain a family teacher and adviser—the sheer rapidity of advance of knowledge renders some specialization inevitable. These organizational changes affect the education of students, as well as creating a need for advanced courses for intending specialists.

With numbers swelling, functions widening, status rising and organization changing it is hardly surprising that the whole post-nursing education of student health visitors has been revolutionized in recent years. The duration of the post-basic course has risen from 6 months to an academic year (in the 1950's) and then to a calendar year (in 1966), and further extension is likely. Sanitary and environmental relics in the training syllabus have been jettisoned, and more and more time devoted to psychology, sociology, social medicine, health education and skills of health visiting. Formal lectures have been reinforced by seminars, discussions, group and individual projects and family studies. Qualified health visitor tutors have been appointed for all courses, and a new grade of field-work instructors has been created. Not least important, academic as well as professional entry standards have become obligatory and techniques of selection of candidates have been improved. For these sweeping developments some credit must go to the Royal College of Nursing: the setting up of the advanced course for the health visitor tutor's qualification in 1948 and of the parallel course in public health nursing administration were big landmarks. Some credit must go to the Health Visitors' Association (formerly named the Women Public Health Officers' Association) and the Scottish Health Visitors' Association, both of which have campaigned for better professional education and have consistently emphasized the importance to the community of an adequate and well-equipped force of health visitors. A great deal of credit must go to the Standing Conference of Health Visitor Training Centres, containing representatives of all training courses and meeting in the offices of the Ministry of Health: it has exerted—and still exerts—on health visitor education an influence of almost incalculable benefit. The greatest share of the credit must, however, be allocated to the Council for the Training of Health Visitors, established under the Health Visitors and Social Work (Training) Act, 1962. During the first 4 years of its existence this statutory body has instituted academic as well as professional entry standards (although in fairness it should be mentioned that well before 1962 some training schools already demanded the equivalent of university entrance); has reorganized both the course syllabus and the examination; has specified a minimum tutor/student ratio; has secured the appointment of field-work instructors; and has completely modernized the post-nursing education of student health visitors. Simultaneously the Council's advisory committees for Scotland and Northern Ireland have successfully tackled some of the problems of health visiting in these countries. All these changes contribute to the urgent need for a new book.

Fifthly, there have been other exciting developments of which two may be chosen for mention here. (a) The setting up by Glasgow Health and Welfare Department and Glasgow University jointly — with the university portion later transferred to the University of Strathclyde — of an advanced mental health course for selected health visitors, producing workers who in large measure combine the skills of health visitors and psychiatric social workers: the course has been described by the Scottish Association for Mental Health as "the most important social development in recent years". (b) The establishment by Aberdeen Health and Welfare Department in 1961 of a course for registered male nurses with an appropriate further qualification to equip them as "male health visiting officers" — a circumlocution employed because, until the law is altered, a man, no matter how well qualified, cannot legally be called a health visitor. The use of men for health education of older boys and young men, for mental after-care and for work with the elderly, has appealed to many local health authorities; courses of preparation are now conducted in London as well as Aberdeen, and it seems likely that in another dozen years between 6 and 10 per cent of health visitors will be men.

Again, although health visiting is more than applied nursing, applied teaching, applied psychology and applied sociology, advances in each of these fields have had repercussions on health visiting, as have developments overseas.

Finally, but by no means least, in the last two dozen years health visiting has acquired a considerable professional literature. Until a distinguished British health visitor tutor, Miss Margaret McEwan, published her *Textbook of Health Visiting* in 1951, and until an equally distinguished American public health nurse, Professor Ruth Freeman, issued her *Public Health Nursing Practice* in 1950, the literature of health visiting was virtually nonexistent. What little had been produced was almost wholly the work of members of other professions. In recent years, by contrast, there has been a flood of articles and papers by members of the profession. The advanced student, specializing in one branch of health visiting, has time to study originals. The general student lacks the time: she needs something that condenses and summarizes the main conclusion.

These, then, are seven reasons why this short book is required.

Why Written by Present Authors?

If a sprinkling of outstanding health visitors qualify as health visitor tutors and thereafter devote their professional lives to the post-basic education of successive groups of students, it is natural that they should include in their number the authors of the appropriate textbooks, just as in the parallel field of social medicine it is natural that the textbooks should emanate from those doctors who have become professors or lecturers in that subject.

The special claim of the health visitor tutors working in the University of Surrey to produce a book on health visiting is fivefold. Firstly, Battersea Polytechnic or Battersea College of Technology—the precursor of the University—was the institution that first started a formal course of training for intending health visitors in 1907. Secondly, the same institution in 1957 was the first to initiate integrated courses in general nursing, health visiting and home nursing. Thirdly, in 1966 the University of Surrey instituted an internal Diploma in the Principles and Practice of Health Visiting. Fourthly, it was the first university in Britain to offer—in 1966—a combined course leading to a nursing qualification and an honours degree in human biology. And fifthly, for many years the Polytechnic (to use its old name) has trained more student health visitors than any other two centres added together.

If a sixth reason is required, it is supplied by the sheer merit of the book.

The Purpose of the Book

As already indicated, this short book in no way seeks to replace textbooks of inter-professional interest: it will not relieve the student of the need to study psychology, sociology, principles of teaching and social medicine. It has, however, been written by experienced health visitor tutors expressly to meet the needs of student health visitors in respect of the principles, methods and techniques of health visiting.

While fully conscious that I possess neither qualification nor practical experience in health visiting, and that I am therefore not really competent to assess the value of the book, I nevertheless venture to express the opinion that it will be of very great benefit to three groups of readers: first, the people for whom it was primarily written, nurses (female or male) entering upon a course for student health visitors; second, qualified health visitors seeking to refurbish their weapons for the battle for better community mental and physical health; and third, some students in allied fields, for example doctors studying for the diploma in public health and social science students with an interest in health and in the work of their future health visiting colleagues. To these groups of potential readers I very cordially recommend *The Principles and Practice of Health Visiting*.

2. The History of Health Visiting

Rosemary Hale

HEALTH VISITING as a service entered its second century in 1962. Like the majority of our social services it began as a local effort of a few voluntary workers attempting to deal with, and bring attention to, a particular need.

Before the close of the eighteenth century Britain could be truly described as a pastoral land. As late as 1800 only London had over 100,000 population. Of the 11,000,000 population of Britain less than 200,000 lived in units of 20,000 or over. Between the years 1801–60 there arose a predominantly urban civilization. Sudden mushrooming of towns occurred mainly in the Midlands and north with scant consideration for the health or comfort of those having to live in them. There came a surge of countrymen deprived of their living due to mechanization and industrial growth, and Irish immigrants to the growing iron works, mines, and cotton factories. By 1850 towns contained about 50 per cent of the people in Britain. Working conditions in factories were bad and infection was common, but living conditions were appalling and remained so, long after factory conditions had begun to improve. To give examples from reports of that period, in Liverpool 40,000, approximately a fifth of the population, existed in cellars. To quote G. M. Trevelyan in *English Social History*:

> These pioneers of "progress" (the slum Landlords) saved space by crowding families into single rooms or thrusting them underground into cellars saving money by the use of cheap and insufficient building material, and by providing no drains — or, worse still, by providing drains that oozed into the water supply.

In Manchester there is report of 1500 cellars where three persons shared one bed and a further 1019 cellars where four or more people shared one bed. Sanitation was often nonexistent, in one area of Manchester there were two privies for 250 people. There were no municipal or national health services until the 1848 cholera epidemic scared the nation into a form of sanitary self-defence.

These conditions, with the consequent dreadful effects on the life and health of the most vulnerable members of the population, i.e. young children, led to the activities of the first small group of women, the pioneers of the present Health Visiting Service. As in all eras of British history where crises occur or needs of the people are exposed, various organizations were formed to attempt to alleviate ignorance, poverty, overcrowding, filth and disease through political reform and other efforts. One such organization was the Manchester and Salford Sanitary Reform Association founded in 1852 with aims to give information that the poor could use with advantage and to aid the infirm and enfeebled. Its female section, the Ladies Reform Association, had as its objects the popularization of health knowledge and "the elevation of the people physically, socially, morally and religiously". In 1862 after a period of distribution of pamphlets which had not produced results the Association decided to employ "a respectable working woman" to pay day-to-day visits among the poor, to teach, and to help. The duties included:

Teaching Hygiene and Child Welfare
They must carry with them carbolic powder, explain its use and leave it where it is accepted; direct the attention of those they visit to the evils of bad smells, want of fresh air, impurities of all kinds; give hints to mothers on feeding and clothing their children.

Social Support
Where they find sickness, assist in promoting comfort of the invalid by personal help.

Teaching of Mental and Moral Health
They must urge the importance of cleanliness, thrift and temperance on all possible occasions.

Later when health clinics or schools for mothers began to appear they were expected to persuade mothers to attend meetings for talks and discussions.

Attempts at home visiting in the interest of children had been made before this, when a dispensary for the infant poor was opened in Red Lion Square, Holborn, in 1769 by Dr. G. Armstrong and home visiting was suggested, but this project was short-lived. Another dispensary was opened in London by Dr. J. B. Davis and it is reported that home visitors were used in connection with this in 1816. In 1859 the New York Infirmary for women and children appointed a "sanitary visitor" and her duties were described as follows: "To give simple, practical instruction to poor mothers on the management of infants and the preservation of the health of their families." About that time William Rathbone had introduced in Liverpool a scheme whereby the city was divided into eighteen districts, each with a nurse, and a "lady visitor". The former for home nursing and the latter for elementary health education and social work.

Why, then, do we consider that the real origin of health visiting was the Manchester and Salford scheme of 1862. One reason is that it succeeded and expanded. In the first 28 years, during which time six of the staff of the voluntary association were transferred to the Manchester Public Health Department to become the earliest health visitors employed by a local authority, the number of visitors on the Association's books rose to fourteen. The second reason is that from the start it was visualized that the health visitor was to be a health teacher and social counsellor rather than a nurse. Florence Nightingale made an emphatic statement in 1891 in line with the association's policy.[*1]

> It seems hardly necessary to contrast sick nursing with this [i.e. health visiting].... The needs of home health bringing require different but not lower qualifications, and are more varied.... She [i.e. the health visitor] must create a new work and a new profession for women.

Florence Nightingale, a pioneer in health education whose written word is still more progressive than many present day health personnel, worked vigorously for the recognition of health visitors or "health missioners" as she called them.

Manchester in 1890 was the first local authority to employ unqualified health visitors and within 2 years of this Florence Nightingale had persuaded the North Buckinghamshire Technical Education Committee to start a course of a sixteen-lecture syllabus in one of their education establishments. Most of the lectures and class discussions were taken by a medical officer, and a general practitioner of the rural areas. Students were taken to visit the homes and written work was undertaken by the students. Sixteen women were selected for this course, twelve remained to take the examination, but only six passed and obtained a certificate. This result is more likely to be due to Florence Nightingale's strict and high standards rather than incapacity of the students. This was the first attempt of a training for health visiting, but we have no record that any further course was conducted in Buckinghamshire. In 1892 Buckinghamshire County Council appointed three of the successful women of the above course as whole-time health visitors to carry out for the first time health visiting in rural areas. Worcester County Council appointed five "lady health missioners" in 1897 for the purpose of giving home instruction in the care of children.

So far no reliable system existed whereby the health visitors could know where new babies were. It was a statutory requirement under the Births and Deaths Registration Act, 1874, to register a birth before the infant was 6 weeks old, but no provision existed to pass on such information to medical officers of health, and in any case serious illness and death could occur before a visit could be paid. For the purpose of visiting some local authorities paid a fee for the registrar to send a weekly list of registered births. The London County Council progressed further in their capacity as local supervising authority under the Midwives Act,

1902, by arranging that midwives notified births to the medical officer of health of the metropolitan borough in which the infant was domiciled.

By 1905 fifty areas of Britain had health visitors or lady sanitary inspectors. Here we must pay tribute to Dr. S. G. H. Moore, Medical Officer of Health of Huddersfield and the Huddersfield Corporation. Having made an intensive study of infant mortality, Dr. Moore commenced a scheme aimed at its reduction. His aim was that mothers of infants should be visited in their own homes by experts to help the mother nurse the infant herself. In 1905 Huddersfield Corporation appointed two assistant medical officers to work as health visitors. In addition to these salaried officers eighty volunteer health visitor members of Huddersfield Public Health Union worked in the wards of the town with a lady superintendent to arrange the work in each district. To encourage notification of births one shilling was paid for each notification to the Medical Officer of Health, within 24 hours of births. Each home was then visited for the purpose of giving guidance on infant management. It is significant that Dr. Moore emphasized that visits must be for the health of the baby only and not to dispense charity, that visits should be entirely optional on the part of those visited and that the visiting should be paid in earliest days of life.[*2] These are important principles of health visiting even today. To further the establishment of this service the Huddersfield Corporation Act was passed in 1906 which required notification of births in Huddersfield. This proved so successful that the notification of Births Act, 1907, was passed; this was a permissive Act and only applied to areas where it was adopted. In 1915 another Act made notification of births compulsory for the whole country; thus, the most important basis for health visiting was laid.

By the turn of the century it was being realized that a health visiting service had great possibilities in helping to reduce infant mortality and morbidity. Serious consideration of suitable professional training was emerging. The attempt in Buckinghamshire to provide a special training appears not to have been repeated and where health visitors were employed the majority had no professional training, some had medical qualifications, some were female sanitary inspectors. By 1907 at least two courses to prepare women for the profession of health visiting had begun, at Bedford College for Women, and Battersea Polytechnic in South West London (now the University of Surrey) had commenced two courses: a 2-year course in the physical and social sciences for educated women without previous qualifications, and a 6-months course for nurses. The Polytechnic issued its own diploma to successful students of these courses and continued to do so for some years after a national certificate was approved. It is relevant to add here that in its pioneering role the Battersea Polytechnic, as the Battersea College of Technology, commenced in 1957 the first course for integrating the training for general nursing, district nursing and health visiting in cooperation with the Hammersmith Hospital and the Queen's Institute of District Nursing. Further, as the University of Surrey, the same establishment in 1966 became the first university to offer an internal Diploma in the Principles and Practice of Health Visiting.

The Royal Sanitary Institute, later renamed the Royal Society for the Promotion of Health, was founded in 1876. It established an examination for inspectors of nuisances, later renamed sanitary inspectors, now public health inspectors. In 1899 an examination in hygiene for school teachers was established, in 1908 the Institute carried out its first examination for health visitors and school nurses. The R.S.I. fostered courses to prepare for this examination and for many years conducted a course in health visiting at its own headquarters. The Institute was later established as the examining body for the health visitor's certificate approved by the Board of Health. Later the R.S.I. was to become the central examining body for a statutory and national certificate in health visiting which responsibility it carried out until 1965 when the Council for the Training of Health Visitors assumed the responsibility.

London was the first authority to demand suitable professional qualifications for health visiting. The London County Council (General Powers) Act, 1908, empowered sanitary authorities to appoint women health visitors. The Health Visitors' (London) Order, 1909, made by the Local Government Board, laid down the qualifications in the London area. The order required that the qualification should be one of the following: (a) a medical degree; (b) full nurse training; (c) the Certificate of the Central Midwives Board; (d) some nurse training and the Health Visitor's Certificate of an organization approved by the Board; (e) previous duties in local authority service.

In 1916 the medical officer of the Local Government Board recommended that health visitors should have two of the three following qualifications: nurse training, a sanitary inspector's certificate, and the Certificate of the Central Midwives Board. Useful as these qualifications appeared to be it was soon apparent that the work required of health visitors was not being achieved. Furthermore, it was only in the London area that any special qualifications were demanded and as could be expected the standard of work throughout the country was very variable.

The Maternity and Child Welfare Act which was passed in 1918 gave local authorities powers to organize welfare work. These powers were permissive but in those areas where schemes developed the need for more health visitors was soon apparent. At this time more than 3000 health visitors of various qualifications and standards were employed in Britain. In a report of the Local Government Board at this time it was stated that it regarded health visiting as "the most important element in any scheme for maternity and child welfare".[3]

In 1919 health visiting was formerly established as a profession: the newly formed Ministry of Health and the Board of Education jointly promulgated an official scheme for training health visitors and the Board of Education (Health Visitors Training). Regulations were passed. The Scottish Board of Health adopted a similar scheme. From this time entry qualifications for health visiting could be obtained in three ways: (a) by one-year, post-basic training for trained nurses (no midwifery qualification was required at this time); (b) a different one-year training for a person already a university graduate; (c) a 2-year training (later extended to $2\frac{1}{2}$ years, the first 6 months to be spent in hospital) for a person neither a nurse nor a graduate.

To this time no midwifery training was required but in 1925 the Ministry of Health required that in future midwifery training was to be required for all health visitors and the 1-year health visitor training was reduced to not less than 6 months, to allow for 6 months' midwifery, thus weakening the social and preventive training of the health visitor. This concentrated attention on the maternity and child welfare aspects of the work with necessary and immediate beneficial effects held ultimate danger for the developing profession of health visiting. The 2-year course for health visiting was still an approved training where midwifery but not nursing training was required. This 2 years' training with its emphasis on social and preventive care and the principles of teaching, rather than care, had undeniable advantages. However, this training attracted less and less candidates compared with the 6 months course, and an increasing number of local authorities were showing preference for the health visitor with a nursing training, and gradually through lack of support the 2-year training became obsolete. Later, when midwifery was divided into parts one and two, the first part only was acceptable for future health visitors and some years later an approved 3 months obstetric course within the nurses general training was accepted as an alternative to midwifery training, and it appears this course is an improvement on Part I Midwifery for potential health visitors.

In 1928 the Ministry of Health required all future appointments to health visiting to hold the health visitor's certificate.

As there was no financial scheme the cost of training deterred many candidates from entering. Because of this two schemes were introduced:

(a) An advance of salary during training. In this scheme the candidate undertook to serve as a health visitor for not less than 6 months following training during which time she repaid the advance of salary.

(b) A probationary health visitor scheme by which candidates are appointed by local authorities and paid a proportion of the minimum of a health visitor's salary during training and required to give a period of service after training.

Modified forms of both of these have persisted to the present time and the majority of students are financed under the sponsoring system, the successor of the probationary scheme. Others are financed by various scholarship awards or education awards. A disadvantage of the sponsoring system is that, in addition to the requirement of a period of service following qualification, some local health authorities lay down certain conditions for students during the year of study including how vacations should be used. Fortunately this is a decreasing practice as those responsible for the student's training assume more control.

In 1929 the Local Government Act issued statutory rules and orders, setting out qualifications required of certain officers of the public health team, among them health visitors and tuberculosis visitors, which qualifications are now incorporated in the National Health Service Act, 1946 (Qualifications of Health Visitors and Tuberculosis Visitors, Regulations, No. 1415):

> Any person employed as a health visitor must be a woman who:
> (1) Has been qualified prior to 5th July 1948 to hold the appointment of health visitor; OR
> (2) Has obtained the Health Visitors' Certificate of The Royal Sanitary Institute, under conditions approved by the Minister; OR
> (3) Has obtained the Health Visitors' Certificate issued by The Royal Sanitary Institute of Scotland.

> Any person employed as a tuberculosis visitor must be a woman who:
> (1) Is qualified as a health visitor; OR
> (2) Has been qualified prior to 5th July 1948 to hold the appointment of tuberculosis visitor; OR
> (3) Is a nurse whose name is entered on the general part of the register kept under the Nurses Registration Act 1919, or on the list kept under Section 18 of the Nurses Act 1943, and has had at least three months experience at a sanatorium or hospital, for the treatment of tuberculosis or at a tuberculosis dispensary.

Since 1965 the Certificate of the Royal Society of Health has been replaced by the Certificate of the Council for the Training of Health Visitors.

The control of tuberculosis has been such in recent years that tuberculosis visitors, where such still exist, include other chest conditions in their work. Dispensaries and tuberculosis wards are renamed Chest Units to include all chest conditions.

The minimum period of training was still 6 months but an increasing number of courses extended to 9 months, an academic year, stimulated by an amended and broader syllabus which commenced in 1950 to prepare health visitors for their function envisaged in the National Health Service Act. By 1965, when it was compulsory that health visitor training was to extend over a calendar year, i.e. three terms of theory and practice followed by not less than eleven weeks' supervised practice, there were only a very small number of courses of 6 months remaining in existence.

In 1953 because of the shortage of health visitors and because it was necessary to clarify the changed role of health visitors in the National Health Service the Ministers of Health and Education and the Secretary of State for Scotland set up a working party to advise on the proper field of work, and the recruitment and training of health visitors. The report was published in June 1956 and a study of this report is still to be recommended.[*4] Some of the recommendations have been implemented including the setting up of a number of integrated courses of nurse education incorporating basic nursing and health visiting.

Meanwhile, the courses providing training for health visitors were increasing but still very variable in standard.

Great progress was made when in 1948 the Education Department of the Royal College of Nursing started a full-time academic year course for health visitor tutors, later it was strongly recommended but not obligatory that all courses should have a health visitor with the qualification, in charge. It would have been short-sighted to demand that only health visitors with this specific qualification be considered for posts of responsibility in health visitor training, thus closing the door to health visitors of valuable but different preparation, and the years between 1949 and the present have proved the wisdom of this as the possibility of more graduate nurses including public health has become a reality. However, the need remains for preparation in teaching methods and adequate experience in the practice of health visiting for all tutors in charge of health visitor training. Training has undergone a number of changes as the needs of the community changed, not only in subject content but the methods used to educate the students, from formal lectures only, to more seminars, discussions and individual student work. Courses throughout Britain are based in a variety of establishments and under a variety of administration patterns. There are those based on universities, colleges of technology, technical colleges and the Royal College of Nursing, partially or wholly controlled by the education policy of the establishments, or local health authority controlled courses carried out in any of the mentioned establishments or in their own premises.

Some students have the advantage of full student facilities, education methods, staff and status compared with others less advanced and the venue of the course is not necessarily the measurement of standards. At the time of writing this chapter the variety remains and I sincerely hope we shall retain a variation in interpretation and philosophy between the different courses but a great need to set minimal standards for health visitor selection and their training had been obvious to many for some years.

The setting up of a Council for the Training of Health Visitors together with a Council for Training in Social Work under the Health Visiting and Social Work Act (Training), 1962, is the most significant milestone of recent years in the history of health visiting. One chairman and one secretary are appointed for both councils and some council members are mutual. The Council for the Training of Health Visitors which concerns us here consists of representatives of the health visiting profession from the United Kingdom, the medical profession, including medical officers of health and general practitioners, together with representatives from the field of education concerned with health visitor training, the General Nursing Council and appropriate local authorities. The Council appointed experienced health visitors as professional advisors to the Council, and the education and administration for health visiting is represented in these appointments.

The functions of this Council are:

(a) To promote training by seeking to secure suitable facilities for training of persons intending to become health visitors, by approving courses to be attended by such persons, and by seeking to attract persons to such courses;

(b) To secure further provisions for the training of health visitors if it appears adequate provision is not being made;

(c) To conduct or make arrangements for the conduct of examinations in connection with such courses as mentioned above;

(d) To carry out or assist in research into matters relevant to the training of health visitors.

The most important changes which have taken place since the inauguration of the Council are as follows:–

Training of health visitors has been extended to a calendar year. Theory and practice for an academic year is followed by eleven weeks supervised practice.

A syllabus is now in use which should provide a training more in keeping with the present role of health visitors (Appendix 2).

Field-work instructors are to be employed to supervise the practical training of students and to work in close liaison with course tutors. Field-work instructors are specially selected, experienced health visitors with a special short training to equip them for the work.

A new examination procedure in which each training institution arranges and organizes its own examination by appointing a moderating committee, internal examiners and an external examiner approved by the Council for the Training of Health Visitors.

For the oral examination students present four family studies from the six prepared during training and a project or day book. Discussion on this work between the candidate and the external examiner and one internal examiner comprises the oral examination.

A National Certificate to practice health visiting is awarded to all successful candidates notified to the Council by the training institutions following a satisfactory report at the end of the supervised practical block. In addition some universities will award their own diploma or certificate.

A minimal education level has been set for entry to health visitor training which is a General Certificate of Education certificate of not less than five Ordinary Levels or its equivalent. Some training establishments demand stricter and higher entry conditions.

To summarize, health visiting has moved from a voluntary service of mainly untrained workers to a full state service of highly trained professional workers; from concentration on mothers and young children to health education and social advice to all age groups and the family unit; from concentration on physical health and reduction of disease to promotion and maintenance of physical, emotional and social health; finally, from concentration on one social group in the community to offering a service to all social groups.

References

1. Letters from Florence Nightingale on Health Visiting in Rural Districts.
2. *Infant Mortality*, DR. S. G. H. MOORE.
3. *Hygiene and Public Health*, PARKED, L. G. and KENWOOD, H. R. (1917) (Health Ed. 594).
4. Jameson Report, *An Enquiry into Health Visiting* (June, 1956, H.M.S.O.).

Suggested Reading

English Social History, G. M. TREVELYAN (McKay).
The Early History of the Infant Welfare Movement, G. F. McCLEARY (H. K. Lewis).
The Maternity and Child Welfare Movement, G. F. McCLEARY (P. S. King).
Selected Writings of Florence Nightingale, LUCY RIDGELY SEYMER (Macmillan), Chapters VIII and IX.
A Social and Economic History of Britain, PAULINE GREGG (Harrap).
The Social Services of Modern England, PENELOPE HALL (Routledge and Kegan Paul Ltd.).

3. The Function of the Health Visitor and Future Trends

ROSEMARY HALE

UNDER the National Health Service Act health visitors must be employed by all local health authorities for a specific community function.

> Section 24[1] states:
>   It shall be the duty of every local health authority to make provision in their area for the visiting of persons in their own homes by visitors to be called "health visitors", for the purpose of giving advice as to the care of young children, persons suffering from illness and expectant or nursing mothers and as to the measures necessary to prevent the spread of infection.
> Section 79 defines illness as follows: Illness includes mental illness and any injury or disability requiring medical or dental treatment or nursing.

Thus, not only were the title and functions of the health visitor laid down by statute but it closed the chapter in health visiting history in which the sole function of health visitors was concerned with the maternity and child welfare group and in some areas school children.

This chapter will deal with the broad pattern of health visitors' functions; details will be found elsewhere in this book. Normally health visitors are employed by health committees of local health authorities as members of staff of the health and welfare department. Administration of the service varies considerably, but for a fully effective service giving satisfaction to the public and the health visiting staff, they should be represented and their work co-ordinated by a senior experienced member of their own profession directly responsible to the medical officer of health. The senior health visitor would be expected to concern herself with policy-making where it affected the public health nursing service, at all levels.

Health visitors being highly trained professional women should be free to use their initiative in work where initiative is so essential, therefore the best service will be obtained in a working structure free from rigidity and where those responsible for policy have kept in step with changes and fully understand the present training and function of health visitors.

The Team

For far too long health visitors have worked in isolation, the reason being that health visiting is one of the oldest of family services and for many years the visitors accepted work and responsibilities for which no other service existed. Now an increasing number of specialist workers all concerned with some aspect of family health and welfare are being trained and employed. Team work is essential, not only to provide job satisfaction for all the specialists concerned, and a satisfactory service which is paid for by the public, but also to conserve skilled personnel, most of whom are in short supply, and to avoid wasting the time of the public in repetitive work. The team with which health visitors will normally work includes the family doctors, domicillary midwives, district nurses, teachers and various professional social workers, e.g. psychiatric social workers, child care officers and mental welfare officers.

The team most intimately concerned with family care in health and illness consists of the family doctor, midwife, health visitor and district nurse, therefore on this group rests the responsibility of good liaison with others where their help is needed. Health visitors bear special responsibility as they have the most consistent contact with normal families before any need for other help emerges. Full team work will only be obtained when all concerned know and understand the professional training and functions of their colleagues.

Patterns of Work

Whereas the basic functions of health visitors will obtain in all local authority areas, there exists a considerable variation in patterns and conditions of work. This is inevitable if a service is provided on assessment of need and suitability for the area to be served. This should be understood by those who plan schemes to be applied to areas of this very diverse and variable island.

Let us look at some patterns of health visiting service in this country. In some rural areas the combined work of health visitor and district nurse operates successfully, in which case the public health nurse must be a qualified health visitor. Sometimes domiciliary midwifery is added and the term *generalized work* is applied. Such a combination ceases to be practical when the population density and work load renders it impossible to give adequate time to all nursing and health visiting duties: naturally the needs of the sick must be met first, and the long-term health and preventive work can so easily suffer. However, let us not underestimate the valuable work undertaken in areas where generalized duties are carried out. In some areas where a temporary or permanent special need exists, specialist health visitors may be employed, for example to visit the aged or the handicapped.

Where such specialist health visitors work it is essential that they maintain close liaison with the general health visitors. Ideally all health visitors are family visitors with a workable family load and a geographical area of a size to allow her to carry out all health visiting duties. An increasing number of local health authorities are appointing full-time health education organizers, some of whom are health visitors. Such colleagues are of great assistance in planning, providing equipment for group and exhibition health education. Two other grades of health visitors are being trained and employed in many areas.

Field-work instructors, mentioned in the previous chapter, must be employed wherever student health visitors are to receive practical training. These health visitors remain in practice on a reduced family load. Their work entails close liaison with the tutor of the health visitor course from which her students come. This grade could be the first promotion step towards full-time teaching in health visitor training.

Group advisers. Experienced health visitors selected for special training to function at field level between the general duties, staff and central administration. Whilst still functioning as a health visitor in a greatly reduced area the group adviser acts as support and guide to inexperienced and newly appointed health visitors. As consultant to other health visitors on problematic situations where other specialist help may not be required, the group adviser can organize local case conferences and other forms of team work. Where a group adviser is based in a central clinic she may be responsible for the co-ordination of the work of the centre, including overall organization of health education.

Another important function could be the planning of programmes for students, other than health visitor students, and to receive local visitors.

The functions mentioned here have been done, and still are being carried out in many areas by senior health visitors designated as area nursing officers, or in some cities, centre superintendents. Some, but not all of these will have received additional training in administration. Now it is recognized that whatever the designation, special preparation is needed. The grade discussed here could be considered a first step in promotion towards senior administration.

Lecturer or tutor in charge of health visitor training. This grade of health visitor has been mentioned in a previous chapter. In the structure she ranks as a parallel colleague to the principal or county nursing officer, and their close co-operation is essential to health visitor training. Tutors are responsible for the organization, co-ordination of, and appropriate teaching in health visitor courses. One of their most important functions is the key role in student selection, thus protecting the profession, and the course, against lowered standards. Increasingly health visitor lecturers or tutors are being appointed as members of the academic staff of universities or other education establishments where courses are based, rather than on the staff of a local health authority, as the majority were in the past.

Function

From 1948 health visitors have been responsible for health promotion and social advice to the family as a whole, and the full age range of the community. Where necessary in the interests of family health, they support, and give guidance in cases of illness or handicap in co-operation with the family doctor and hospital staff. The latter responsibility is not a threat to the work of district nurses who are responsible for home nursing care, but gives recognition to a fact, well known and acted upon, by many health visitors before 1948, that in some cases of illness or handicap the health and well-being of the whole family may be involved. Many difficulties could be prevented by the right kind of support, health guidance, and referral to other services. Since 1948 health visitor training has been slowly changing to equip for this broader function, culminating in the improved training and examination patterns from 1965 which provides for the fact that health visitors are involved in physical, emotional and social health promotion, the social aspects of disease and early detection of deviation from the normal. Improvements in basic nurse education of recent years has contributed to this more adequate training.

For social advice and social action to be effective it is necessary for a family or individual to accept and use the health guidance offered; the two functions are indivisible. To give two examples: guidance in dietary needs to an aged person could be valueless without assessment of financial resources, and where necessary, referred for assistance; where a child's normal development is threatened by circumstances the health visitor must take what social action she considers necessary to avert the danger which could mean referral to another colleague or department. Health visitors are in the unique position of being the only professional workers prepared for and specifically employed to take health education into the homes of the public; they are the only regular visitors to homes where there are children of all age groups, and to others such as the elderly. Therefore they are in the position to observe the normal family as a unit before obvious need exists. This places upon health visitors not only the responsibility to promote good health but of detecting at an early stage any deviation from the normal in child development, family relationships, or individual needs of any age group and also to encourage the acceptance of any specialist help necessary and to continue to support the family.

Without wishing to detract from the importance of the health visitors' role with other age groups, it should be emphasized that the education of parents of young children in the essential needs for healthy physical, emotional and social development remains their most important work, and in which they are the key workers. This function is emphasized because on this rests the foundation of family and individual health in its broadest sense. Healthy family life is the basis of a healthy community. Whatever changes occur in health visitor functions in the future, time must be adequate to do this important long-term work properly.

For a multiplicity of reasons including the work of health visitors, the physical health of children has improved and child mortality and morbidity have been greatly reduced, and most dangerous infections controlled. However, there remains **great** need for improvement in mental health and with knowledge and **opportunities** now available to health visitors, there is scope and urgency for guidance to parents in particular, and others, in this aspect of health education.

With improved standards and opportunities in general education and the growing volume of literature and other forms of education in child care, and health education for all, it may appear that health visitors are superfluous in this field. In practice the need is greater than ever before because many, whose need may be greatest, read little of the authentic health guidance, and what is seen of any value on television is rarely applied by the viewers to their own situation, and the absence of interpretation and discussion is an obvious drawback. Those who read from even the most reliable sources of health education soon find apparently conflicting ideas particularly in child development and care, causing considerable anxiety to some parents. To these the personal guidance, interpretation and reassurance of the health visitor is valuable. Furthermore, the most effective help is that assessed on individual or local needs and their capacity to use it. This is as true of education as any other forms of service. Of growing importance is the role health visitors must be prepared to play in the health needs of other groups, such as the aged, and families with a handicapped member, needing their particular assessment and support.

Assistance in the screening and testing for early detection deviation from the normal in homes, schools and centres is an important part of the preventive work of health visitors. All this, rightly within the sphere and competence of health visitors, is time-consuming. The problem of too few health visitors, with the consequent too heavy family load for the majority, remains, and will not be easy to overcome. Particularly as it is essential that never again in the name of expediency must the standard of candidates, or training, for the profession, be allowed to fall.

The skills of health visitors must be conserved for the work they are trained and employed to do. More ancillary help is needed in some areas to carry out work not requiring health visiting training or skills. Health visitors themselves must be prepared to continuously review the work they are doing and to delegate work which does not require their personal attention; also to refer to other colleagues, work, often of a long-term intensive nature, requiring a specialized professional training, and skills of a different kind.

Other ways of conserving time and energy of professional personnel have been pointed out in Ministry of Health circulars[1] to local authorities 26/59 and 12/65 dealing with ancillary help, adequate transport, etc. Added to this could be improved communication, including the need for all professional workers to have direct contact with each other.

Future Trends

According to the philosophy of Heraclitus nothing is ever static, if there is not progression there is regression. To justify its existence and retain its usefulness a profession which gives a public service must change as needs change. The health visiting profession has had many changes, more are in sight and doubtless there are others around the corner. This chapter will deal with a few of the obvious changes.

The first and perhaps the most important trend which is gaining momentum is the closer working liaison with family doctors. Important pioneering work has been carried out for several years, and highly successful team work can be observed in a number of local health authority areas. The family doctor and health visitor are two key workers for the health and welfare of the family, providing together a fuller and more effective service because their functions are complementary. The doctor provides diagnosis, treatment, and general medical care, with the assistance of his other two colleagues, the midwife and district nurse. The health visitor provides social assessment, necessary action and health guidance to alleviate or prevent family and individual stress, and in the case of the aged and handicapped, to prevent further deterioration in the social situation by provision of supporting services, particularly in those homes where routine nursing care by a trained district nurse is not required. The health visitor can supply in the homes of the doctor's practice, health education where it is most needed, and in an acceptable form. Working with the family doctor provides the health visitor with opportunities of contact with a wider clientele, of particular importance being the middle-aged of both sexes, the aged and handicapped, at a stage earlier than hitherto when supportive and preventive measures can be more effective. Thus the health visitor is enabled to extend her work in care and after-care, as was envisaged in the National Health Service Act. The first priority work of health promotion with parents and children in normal homes will be strengthened by this partnership, by the removal of real or imagined conflict of advice, and the confidence families would have in such a team. The value of this trend must be so obvious that the administrative and other problems now existing in some areas will diminish, particularly as more doctors and health visitors with a broader and more satisfactory professional training come on the scene.

Male Health Visitors

Health visiting has been and still is a female profession. However, there are signs that this situation will change in the near future. A lead has been given in Aberdeen by Dr. Ian MacQueen and Miss D. J. Lamont, Principal Tutor to the Aberdeen Health Visitor Course. In 1961 they commenced an experiment in training a small number of suitable male nurses as male health visiting officers. Entry conditions were as for female candidates, with the exception of a midwifery or obstetric qualification, an additional qualification which male nurses could not offer; the acceptable alternatives to be a qualification in psychiatric nursing or district nursing. The course is run simultaneously with the female health visitor course and in large measure is identical with it. The examination is of the same standard as that for female health visitors. Reports suggest that male nurses, so prepared, are a valuable addition to a health visiting staff. Dr. MacQueen suggested a ratio of seven men to a hundred women as practicable, but it is doubtful that this number on a national scale will ever be available. The functions already undertaken by some of the Aberdeen health visiting officers could be a pattern for future male health visitors, for example health education to those groups now often neglected, such as schoolboys, male adolescents and male clubs. Female health visitors would sometimes welcome the assistance of an equal male colleague with some fathers not amenable to female guidance, although such fathers are normally few in a health visitor's area, they constitute an important group. Mental health after-care, particularly where the patient is a male, could be a fruitful field of work and has already proved to be. In some areas general and specialist health visitors are already doing valuable mental after-care work, in co-operation with mental welfare colleagues and local hospitals. Care of the male aged and handicapped could be another valuable field of work for male health visitors, for which their nurse and health visitor training could adequately prepare them. Male health visitors could prove particularly valuable in assisting their colleagues in organization and teaching of health education to groups of the public.

Apart from some of the maternal and child welfare functions there is no reason why male health visitors should not find a place in all aspects of health visiting.

Administrative Changes

The indications are that changes may soon take place in the administrative structure within which health visitors' work as reorganization of local authorities and the social services takes shape. The department from which health visitors' work is not of great importance so long as in any future pattern they find their rightful place in the team providing comprehensive community care where their full contribution can be used, and a vigilant profession must see that this obtains.

Health Education

There are also indications that major changes in the provision of health education to the public are being planned, some in accordance with the Cohen Report.[2] Health visitors, themselves health educators, must be prepared to co-operate fully in future schemes. The present training for health visitors provides a more adequate preparation for health education and on a wider range of subjects than was once considered their sphere of education. To give one important example, groups, particularly womens groups, are now asking for information on cancer and some health visitors are playing an important part in cancer education, individually or as part of a scheme. This is a hopeful trend and one in which health visitors should play an important part in co-operation with their doctor colleagues.

Preparation for the Future

Major changes in the training of health visitors have recently taken place but no healthy profession is ever fully satisfied. An adequate supply of nurses of suitable calibre depends on the policy of basic nurse education and it is a matter of some importance to health visiting that the entry to our profession at basic nursing level should not be less than is now required at health visitor training level, then perhaps we shall see a reduction in the time needed for basic nursing education with more time available for post-basic experience and specialized training of which health visiting will be one.

This chapter will end with a quotation which could well be the prayer of all health visitors: "God give us the courage to change those things that can and ought to be changed; the serenity to accept those things we cannot change; the wisdom to see the one from the other."

References

1. Ministry of Health, Circulars 26/59, 12/65.
2. *Cohen Report on Health Education*, H.M.S.O., 1964.

Suggested Reading

An Inquiry into Health Visiting, Ministry of Health, Department of Health for Scotland, and Ministry of Education, H.M.S.O.

First Report of the Council for the Training of Health Visitors, 1962–1964. From Clifton House, Euston Road, London, N.W.1.

The Health Visitor and the Family Doctor. Reprinted from the *Journal of the College of General Practitioners*, 1961, vol. IV, 304. Available from the Royal College of Nursing.

4. The Skills in Health Visiting Practice

A. THE ART AND SKILL OF INTERVIEWING

ROSEMARY HALE

GOOD interviewing is as essential to effective health visiting as to any other form of social work. Although much of health visiting interviewing consists of assessment for health counselling, the health visitors work will often be involved with more complex interviews, and the continuous use of therapeutic interviewing to relieve stress.

The principles in this book are concerned with the practical, and the less tangible aspects involved in verbal, and non-verbal, interaction between persons working toward a common goal.

Much of what is written can be applied to any professional interviewing. Because all interviewing is founded on common principles, some will have particular relevance to the practice of health visiting. Whereas the interviewing process can involve more than two persons, the subject matter here will be chiefly concerned with the face to face two person interviewing, in which health visitors are involved in homes, offices, centres, or schools. Throughout, the term client will be used, rather than interviewee, which appears to be the least cumbersome of two un-attractive designations.

In contrast to ordinary conversation an interview is planned, purposeful conversation with an objective in mind.

The objectives in health visiting would include; to help insight and gain knowledge, to further understanding toward working relationships, to assess needs, to arrive at appropriate action and to relieve stress and give reassurance, this latter being perhaps one of the most important of the less tangible aspects of the preventive measures in health visiting practice.

In interviewing the health visitor must recognize that being a unique individual she can affect her clients by her own attitudes and background.

The capacity to understand individuals and families in terms of their particular culture and attitudes, and how they may differ from her own, is essential for successful interviewing, in fact for effective health visiting practice. We all have a tendency to measure others by the yardstick of our own culture pattern and standards, which if not fully faced and under-stood can be a serious block in interviewing. Therefore any health visitor new to an area needs to study the characteristics of the area, the quality and pattern of family and community life; the key people and important influences of the area. In addition, to study any local health, or social problems. This is slow but essential preparation, not only for interviewing but for the practice of health visiting, and the reason why the unnecessary movement of health visitors is to be deplored. It is so easy to build up a set of superficial and false assumptions about persons and families which is the great enemy in any social work. We are all aware of the peculiar assumptions and generalizations held by persons of one part of this island about those of other areas. An illustration may assist here. A young and recently trained professional worker from an industrial city took a post in a small southern market town. She had retained an image of a near feudal system still at work in such an area and mentally divided the community into the served and the servile. Her clients received her with the greatest courtesy but her social work was far from successful and results poor, she remained a stranger. She had mistaken quiet courtesy for servility and dependence. This points to the importance of the intensive personal work over and above professional training necessary for successful practice, and work satisfaction. In addition to knowledge of standards and culture patterns of her area, a health visitor must know herself, face up to her own personality, standards, and prejudices, which are the results of her background and experience. She needs to be honest with herself in respect of her strengths and her weaknesses, with such self examination, she is less likely to project her own standards on others, the surest way to greater understanding and tolerance. Although a friendly attitude in all interviews is essential, it is important to remember that professional service is being offered. A problem can occur if a professional worker tries to combine a friendship role and a professional relationship in which case both relationships will suffer.

Interviewing Practice

To distinguish an interview from ordinary conversation it is necessary that the health visitor is clear as to the purpose of the interview. A planned pattern is essential, such pattern being capable of modification when necessary as rigidity is not good practice. The late Porter Lee,[1] a teacher in social work practice and in the art of interviewing, listed four elements in the pattern of an interview:
(1) the start; (2) crises in the trend of discussion; (3) psychological movements; and (4) conclusion. Although Lee wrote for social case workers his pattern is relevant to all professional interviewers.

Interviewing Stages

The start or commencement of the interview can set the quality of the whole process particularly if it is the first contact. If an appointment has been made it is important that the interviewer is punctual and that the client is afforded all the courtesies of a guest. In health visiting the majority of interviews will take place in the homes where the health visitor is the guest. She must be prepared to adapt to situations which may occur in any home and sometimes it may be necessary to postpone an important interview to a more appropriate time because there is no merit in pressing on with an interview when circumstances are against any success. From the start it is important that client and interviewer are clear as to the purpose of the interview. The first few moments can be tense and awkward for the client, and this can best be overcome if the interviewer makes sure he is comfortable and for a few minutes engages in general conversation, other than the purpose of the interview. Here an easy, friendly personality is very important together with the environment in which the interview is to be conducted.

The middle phase or trend of the discussion commences at the point when the interview begins to focus on the purpose; and free discussion flows with most of the talking by the client. During this phase psychological blocks and other reasons may check the conversation flow or cause diversions; here the listening, questioning, skills and the sympathetic attitude of the interviewer will be important. Some people find it difficult if not impossible to speak directly of the most painful aspect of their problem.

Disrupting incidents from outside sources may occur during an interview. This is a particular hazard in health visiting in shared or inadequate working accommodation and during home interviews. Details of the interview environment will be discussed later.

The final phase of the interview can take place for one of several reasons:

(1) When a predetermined time period has been set for the interview; in this situation unless it is possible or desirable to prolong the time, the interviewer must recognize the need, in some cases, to make another interview appointment before they part.

(2) When one of the two decided that the purpose for meeting has been achieved, and this will be fairly easy in the majority of less complex health counselling interviews. However, the situation must be treated with reserve in more complicated situations when the client decides to end the interview. Any sign of agitation about time by the interviewer, such as looking at a clock or watch, or any sign of diminution of focused interest can make a sensitive client decide to end an interview pre-

maturely, and confidence in the professional worker may be reduced for any future relationship.

Skills or Techniques in Interviewing

The interviewing process means the overall pattern or structure, and this will be much the same as all interviews. On the other hand, the skills employed within the structure are unique and variable. Blending of the skills, with the unique personality of the interviewer, is called the art of interviewing.

Listening

The ability to listen is the first and most important skill. Effective listening involves not only what is heard in verbal conversation but also what is communicated through pauses, silence, and change of voice. The truly listening ear can often bring greater benefit and comfort than practical help and other services. There is an art in true listening and it is described in the following quotation extract: —

> To be able to listen one should abandon or put aside prejudices, pre-formulations, and daily activities. When you are in a receptive state of mind things can be easily understood, you are listening when your real attention is given to something. But unfortunately most of us listen through a screen of resistance. We are screened by prejudices, our own desires, fears and attitudes.[2]

The components for effective listening can be described as follows.

The first is concentration on the client, active participation which means keeping the mind receptive, alert and flexible for any changes in the client's conversation or attitude. The second is comprehension, and understanding of the true meaning of what we hear rather than what we think we hear. Finally, hearing the person objectively without the screen of our own preconceived opinions and conclusions. To sum up, the art of listening involves hearing all that is said and otherwise expressed and being able to sense important omissions. Listening is not an easy art to master, it takes perseverance and experience but the effect is so worthwhile because successful social relationships and professional work depends on it.

Observation

Health visitors being already trained and experienced nurses will bring to their work an understanding of the importance of detailed observations and in many the skill will be well developed. In interviewing, factors other than what is said can be important and relevant to the situation. If the client is known to the interviewer any change in appearance or manner should be noted. Signs of fatigue, anxiety and tension, here the face, hands and posture will tell the observer much. Self confidence, or lack of it, can often be seen in the manner a client enters a room and sits on a chair. During home visit interviews the health visitor can use her skilled observation to great effect. In homes already known to her any significant changes in standards, or relationships could be of utmost importance. Here a word of warning is necessary. It is so easy to make quick, erroneous assumptions on observed facts, therefore it is essential to reserve initial assumptions until other factors during the interview substantiates or refutes.

Use of Questions

Questioning at all times, whether in social intercourse or during interviews, must be treated with care and reserve. Direct questioning is repugnant to most people and often appears as an intrusion in private affairs, therefore replies will be evasive. Questions have a place in interviewing but how and when to use them is important. Any question which elicits a mere yes or no response, except when that is all that is needed, normally indicates lack of skill of the interviewer. Some forms of questions used in interviewing are as follows.

The restatement question in which what the client has said is returned in slightly different words, can give the client opportunity to assess the meaning and importance of what has been said.

Cross-examination by question has no place in professional interviewing or anywhere in health visitor practice. Such practice shows lack of skill, and an authoritarian attitude. In the same category of undesirable practice is the leading question which often serves to boost the ego of the interviewer rather than help the client.

The "why" question when used to help through to deeper understanding, can be valuable. The "what" question used with skill can encourage the client to discuss any plans he may have made or will make to help himself. For the reticent, anxious client, carefully inserted questions, or expressions of reassurance are necessary to encourage continuation of his narrative.

However, as has already been indicated, not all silences during interview need to be filled in by questions or expressions and knowing when not to interject oneself is as important as good questioning. The interviewer who feels compelled to fill all silences by her own talk is more concerned for her own comfort than desire to help the client. Skill in handling silence and the other skills mentioned here can only be developed by experience in their use, by periodic revaluation of one's methods and results, and continuous effort toward better understanding of people.

Preparation or Setting

The majority of interviews in health visiting take place in homes where special setting would not apply. However, for those interviews more complicated than the routine health counselling, an appointment should be made, convenient to the client when she is free, and ideally at a time when a measure of privacy and non-interruption can be expected. Health visitors must learn to adapt to conducting interviews in far from ideal conditions. When conducting an interview in her office certain factors are worthy of consideration. Interviewing from behind a loaded desk can give the impression of authoritarian power, and shortage of time, so harmful to professional interviews. Seating arrangements should supply comfort, and give an impression of equality and friendliness. This can be achieved in the most unsatisfactory of offices. If the office is shared, important interviews should be arranged elsewhere or when colleagues are out. Sometimes, as in the case of an unmarried working mother, or a man, an evening interview appointment is essential.

Note-taking

Whereas any client would understand the necessity in some cases for occasional notes to be taken, the practice of note-taking during the interview should be reduced to an absolute minimum and wherever possible dispensed with altogether. Note-taking will reduce the concentration and listening necessary on the part of the interviewer, and can reduce the value of the face to face relationships. Apart from this, some clients if aware that much of their conversation is being committed to paper will restrict the amount they expose, a very natural reaction. It is poor practice on the part of health visitors to obviously take written notes whilst home visiting for any reason, and when such practice is necessary, e.g. survey imformation, the client is asked to co-operate and reasons given.

It should be unnecessary to say that "doodling" has no place in interviewing situations, not only because it is a discourteous habit, but can be extremely irritating to clients.

Recording Interviews

Recording as a health visiting skill is dealt with later in this chapter. I shall conclude by saying recording of an interview should be done whilst information and impressions are fresh in the memory. The record should give a clear picture of the client and the situation in logical sequence. Interview records are highly personal and confidential documents and must be treated as such by being kept in locked files and only used in the interest of the client. Some information of a highly confidential nature could only be divulged to a professional colleague with the permission of the client and only when such knowledge was essential to assist the client.

To conclude, interviewing is skilled communication on the part of the interviewer used for the purpose of assessing the most effective action necessary to assist, or, as in health education the real health needs of persons and families, or as a therapeutic measure in cases of stress.

B. RECORDING AND REPORT WRITING

Marion Loveland

Recording

RECORD-KEEPING is an integral part of the work of the health visitor. In order that she undertakes it intelligently and does it willingly, it is necessary that she understands the value and purpose of the records she keeps.

One of the first records the health visitor finds when starting on her work is the birth record card. This card is compiled from the birth notification sent to the medical officer of health. The health visitor must ensure that she has a record card for every child that she visits. This card will be retained in the area in which the child lives for the first 5 years of its life, and will be kept up to date by the health visitor recording each visit she makes to the child. It will be a record of physical, mental, social and environmental progress and serves as a reminder when future visits are undertaken. It is therefore essential that the records are kept up to date and that relevant information is recorded. In many areas this infant record card is sent to the school medical service department for inclusion in the child's school medical records. This information can be of use to the school medical officer, school health visitor and the teaching staff. The question arises as to how much information can be disclosed. The health visitor obtains a great deal of very confidential information during the course of home visiting, which throws light on the health of the family and the individual. The decision to give such information to others must be that in doing so it will be for the good of the family, but it should only be disclosed to bona fide workers who are working with the family.

Record cards properly kept will help the health visitor to plan her work and to know what she has to do at any given time. They should be written legibly and chronologically.

Information collected during home visiting includes:

1. Particulars of ages, sexes and health of the family and any past illness.

2. Environmental conditions, to include numbers of rooms, occupants, cleanliness, sleeping arrangements, etc.

3. Social conditions, such as income of the household, rent paid, any regular payments to be made, etc.

4. Dates and details of home visiting done, any advice or information given.

5. Attendances at clinics, hospitals or general practitioner of any member of the family.

6. Any action taken and the results achieved.

Record cards of this kind are in use for many sections of the community, e.g. expectant mothers, the elderly, the handicapped, etc. In every case the card will provide a record of visits made, of advice given or of help required and help obtained, and the results of any action taken.

Record cards vary all over the country, with the exception of the school medical record card which is universal. Many cards have headings on them which only need to be ringed or underlined; full use should be made of these facilities as it will save time and writing. Many areas also have family record cards or family folders; these should be used when there is a change in the family circumstances. Family and individual progress should be fully reported.

Every health visitor is required to keep a daily record of work and a record of families visited. The method of recording these varies throughout the country and the new health visitor will have to be instructed in the method in use where she is working.

Local health authorities are required to return certain facts and statistics to the Ministry of Health. Local authorities use these figures to present the report on the health of the area and study these figures with others, to guide their policy. They will want to see what use is made of the services provided and to find the needs of their population. This may be a short-term emergency policy, such as in an epidemic or a long-term policy. The local health authority will want to deploy their finances to meet these needs and will also want to ensure that their staff are being used to the best advantage of the community they serve.

In turn the Ministry of Health uses the statistical facts sent to them by local authorities to prepare the Chief Medical Officer's report on the health of the country as a whole and certain areas in particular. In the light of these facts policies are made and money made available to carry them out.

The record cards will be available to other members of the staff and will be there if the health visitor is off sick, retires or moves to another area. The card should form a continuous link between the family and the health visiting service.

Attendances at clinics of all kinds also have to be recorded. Each local authority will have its own method of recording these but it is the health visitor's responsibility to see that these numbers are accurately recorded, particularly where she has delegated the task of recording to a voluntary worker or a clerk.

Records of all kinds should be kept in locking files and should not be destroyed without permission.

Report Writing

During the course of her work the health visitor will be required to write reports. They fill a useful purpose in providing information of a detailed nature in certain situations. Some reports have to be written at regular intervals, such as monthly or quarterly, on certain sections of the community, e.g. the handicapped, the elderly, problem families. Others may be written in response to a request from the medical officer of health, the housing manager, a hospital, etc. Reports can be written when a person or family requests some special consideration, or the health visitor may decide that it is necessary to write a report to draw attention to a certain set of circumstances.

All reports, for whatever purpose, contain certain necessary information, such as name, address, family composition, environmental conditions, which are useful pointers to family life.

Reports of the routine kind are very often written on structured forms which have the same set of questions to be answered and the same information required each time the report is required. There will always be space for the health visitor to express her own opinion and make any recommendations.

When a health visitor is asked for a report on a certain situation she must make sure that she understands why the report is required and she will be given particulars of the situation on which she is to report. Any recommendation asked for must be clearly understood and the health visitor will make her suggestions in the light of the circumstances she finds. She should be prepared to stand by her recommendation and be ready to supply further information if required. Recommendations follow statements of facts given and the health visitor must be prepared to find out all she can. Even if the family is well known to the health visitor, it is sometimes useful to discuss the family with others who may be concerned. So often people interviewed say different things according to their assessment of the importance of the interviewer; they may consider that one person carried a higher status than another and will endeavour to please.

In certain circumstances it may be necessary to inform the client what is going to be recommended but the health visitor must make it clear that others may make the final decision, which will be a fair one.

When the health visitor decides to make a report because of circumstances which do not satisfy her she will not necessarily reveal to the family her intention to do so.

The health visitor must tell the client that the information given will be treated with confidence in so far as possible but that, in order to do the best for the client, others may need to have access to the report.

All reports must be accurate, concise, relevant and written legibly. The health visitor should sign and date reports and keep a copy. She will give at the beginning of any report the relevant social, physical and environmental conditions and the name, address and composition of the family.

The health visitor will expect to be kept informed of any decisions made and will accept them. She may have to adapt her attitudes when any change in the situation occurs. She will keep a record of action taken and results achieved.

Summary

Records
1. Accurate.
2. Relevant.
3. Informative.
4. Legible.
5. Easily accessible for future reference.

Reports
1. Tabulate where possible.
2. Recommendation must be clearly shown.
3. Copies should be kept.
4. Should be signed and dated.
5. Should be addressed to the recipient.

Records and reports should both show action taken and results achieved.

Filing

The filing of reports and records is important.

They should be readily accessible and easily found when required.

Different filing systems are used throughout the country but are usually the same in one local authority area. The health visitor will make herself familiar with the method used in the area where she works.

Records well filed will help the health visitor to plan her work, show her work load at any one time and keep her priorities for visiting continually before her. Cards filed behind month index cards will facilitate this. Normally files are provided for each health visitor which will contain her record cards. Any cards relating to the family will more usefully be kept together, where there are not family folders. Copies of reports should be kept with family cards, or in the family folders, so that at any one time the complete family history can be referred to.

A good, well-kept filing system will ensure that the records are available in the absence of the health visitor for any reason.

Family Studies

The presentation of these family studies is now part of the examination for health visitors. They should bring home to the student the image of the health visitor as the long-term family visitor. The compilation of these studies quickly brings the student into family situations and gives her a measure of independence early in her training. The student should be presented as "a student health visitor" to the families who are the subject of her family studies; she must understand that, if there is anything she is unable to deal with, she will say so and refer back to the field-work instructor for help and advice, never forgetting to make sure that the family is left with an assurance that some action is being taken.

In order that these family studies should be of value in the training of the health visitor student, some guidance must be given to her before she starts to write them.

The following is one suggestion of what might be included, recognizing that the format may vary between different training units.

1. At the beginning of each study, biographical information of each member of the family, to include health record, occupation, etc., and any family separations.

2. Housing situation. Kind of accommodation; house, flat, etc. Ownership of property; owner occupied, council property, etc. Number of rooms used solely by the family and how allocated. Total number of occupants. Observations of the overall comfort and state of the home.

3. Chronological study of the family. If one person is particularly

the subject of the study, e.g. young baby, old person living with the family, handicapped person, etc., a report on this member should be the first entry.

4. A statement of the aims of each visit and how far these aims are achieved should be included.

5. If a statement such as "this child appears to be backward" is made, the reasons for such an assumption should be stated and any action taken recorded.

6. A resume at the end of each family study, of the community services available to the family, and whether used or not.

Apart from the value to the health visitor in practice, family studies are an invaluable instrument of training as a basis of discussion between student and tutors, and the student and field-work instructor.

C. CO-OPERATION AND TEAM WORK

Grace Owen

HUMAN relationships are widely recognized these days as being a very important aspect of any working situation. It is all too easy to dismiss the subject of co-operation in this team work, as being something we all know about, in rather a vague way; after all, as nurses we have been accustomed to working in a team and mixing with different people and performing a variety of roles, and we may well feel we have adequate experience of this skill. Also it is tempting to assess some of the current literature written on this subject as being too theoretical to be of any practical value to a health visitor, who spends most of her time working with people.

However, it should be possible to discover a point of balance between these two approaches, and to find some basic principles which can be applied directly to the working situation of the health visitor, and perhaps help us to clarify our own thinking.

As no health visitor can expect to work in isolation from her colleagues, it is of paramount importance that good co-operation exists, otherwise the family and individuals are going to suffer from disorganized and duplicated services, and there will be waste of valuable time and effort, and loss of efficiency and economy. In any situation where co-operation is essential, if skills can be developed and used it will facilitate the smooth functioning of organization, making for efficiency and good relationships throughout the service, in the long run benefitting the recipient. In addition, if applied to the health visitor's work, it will ensure that she remains a respected colleague among her professional peers.

One of the most important basic principles in any team work, is that each member shall be fully aware of his own role and function in relation to the other members of the team. It is essential for each individual to understand something of the contribution each member makes towards the whole purpose of the team in order to work effectively.

It is not difficult to appreciate how important this is in application to the health visitor's work. She needs to be aware of her own potential and ability to deal with situations, and to do so confidently within her own field, and also needs to accept her limitations, and refer to the appropriate colleague when she finds anything is beyond her sphere.

It follows that she will want to know something of the training and day to day work of those in other disciplines and departments, so that she knows to whom she must refer situations that arise. It also helps to have a working knowledge of the correct procedure for communicating and passing on information.

In an area where good communications are established, co-operation can be efficient, but where few recognized channels exist, and much is left to the individual, a health visitor will do well to ensure that she gets to know the people she needs to contact, so that they can come to a mutual arrangement concerning their methods of communication, and know when and where to contact each other in moments of urgency.

It is desirable that it is possible for workers at field level to be able to contact each other directly, without reference to an intermediary, but at the same time essential that any action decided upon or reports received, should be communicated to the appropriate senior officer (i.e. health visitor superintendent or medical officer of health).

The establishment of good communications through recognized and acceptable channels can be regarded as another basic principle of good team work.

Not only is good communication important on a horizontal level, between field-workers, but vertically throughout the hierarchy of staff. While regulations of this kind may seem irksome, they must be observed to ensure that accurate records are kept, and information reaches its intended destination.

One very elementary principle of good team work which must be mentioned, if only because its importance is often overlooked, is that of courtesy and consideration between members of staff and colleagues. This involves again the prompt communication of information, and also recognition of the accepted practices and codes of other disciplines, even where the reason is not apparent. Telephone conversations can be a source of misunderstanding, if abruptly conducted, and especial care needs to be taken.

Often the health visitor needs to take the initiative in making contact and establishing relationships with her colleagues in other departments. There may be some who are quite unfamiliar with the work of the health visitor in relation to their own clients or patients, and this presents an opportunity for enlightenment, by making the initial approach, explaining her work, offering co-operation and perhaps leaving a card.

When starting work in a new area, it can be a very time-consuming task to make contact will all one's colleagues, but it is interesting and well worthwhile, as first impressions are important, and help to ease the way for further contacts by telephone at a later date. It is much easier to talk with someone who is known as a person, rather than a "voice".

Being an "all purpose" visitor, much of the health visitor's work is inevitably liaison, and having access to so many families, she will be approaching a variety of statutory bodies and social agencies.

At this point we shall discuss some of the specific areas of the health visitor's work where co-operation is likely to be most important. Much of this may be very obvious to any who have already worked in the community, but to students whose experience has been mainly in hospital, it can be helpful to enter community work with some preparation, knowing with whom they will have the closest association.

Obviously the health visitor's most frequent associates will be her own colleagues, with whom she may share office accommodation or a clinic, and in addition may have easy access to members of the administrative staff.

By contrast, in the more rural areas she may be very isolated, and it is then even more important that the channels for good communications exist. Opportunities for her to meet her own contemporaries provide mutual support in an otherwise lonely situation.

Often in urban areas families may be known to several health visitors, where areas adjoin, and children attend school in another area, and the mother visits the ante-natal clinic in yet another hospital over the boundary, and information needs to be shared.

Health visitors who work in a central office or clinic will also have frequent contact with the clinical and administrative staff. As adequate clerical help becomes more readily available, it matters that it should be wisely used in record keeping, filing and correspondence. There may also be voluntary helpers or domestic staff in a welfare centre and they need a very special form of recognition and co-operation.

Other regular contacts within the department will be made with the health visitor administrators, who will be available for consultations, support and encouragement, in the course of their duties in co-ordinating the work of the staff within the area. The health visitor superintendent will need to have a general picture of the staffing situation within her area, and knowledge of any major crises occurring within the community, so that she can assess the needs of her staff.

Each health visitor will have full responsibility for organizing and arranging her own work, with due regard to the fixtures and needs in her area, but it is essential that adequate reports should be passed on so that the superintendent is kept well up to date, as she may at any time be called upon for information.

It will often be necessary to welcome students from hospitals or colleges for a day or two—this may be very time-consuming but should be regarded as an important opportunity to introduce the work to others, who may in future years be in a position where they need the co-operation of a health visitor. Impressions gained in one short visit can affect these future relationships.

Before we leave discussion of the contacts made in the centre for the health visitor based there or making frequent calls, in many urban areas we find there are a number of other local authority services using the same building; and this provides excellent opportunities for good liaison. It is comparatively easy to establish communications when buildings, offices, canteens and kitchens are shared, but the opportunity may be missed through failure to appreciate the work of the other person.

Dental, foot and orthopaedic clinics are examples of those used frequently for referrals. Family planning clinics and child guidance clinics often share the same premises, and in addition to accepting referrals, they offer facilities for their experts to act in a consultative capacity to health visitors who wish to discuss relevant family problems. The Children's Department and the Home Help Service may also be readily available in local offices in towns, but in rural areas much of the contact with other departments will be by telephone, or by arranged contact on the area.

Another sphere where co-operation is very necessary is with local hospital staffs. This may present difficulties in densely populated areas but it is often possible to get to know individual medico-social workers or ward sisters, especially in maternity departments, and come to a mutual arrangement for communication.

The health visitor's function in schools will be fully discussed in a separate chapter, and it is sufficient to say here that co-operation with the school staff, parents and the school medical officer ensures the smooth running of the School Health Service. It is also a significant factor in ensuring that the teachers have a realistic image of the health visitor in relation to school work and can use her in a consultative capacity on any matters relating to the children's health, welfare or health education. This will only occur if the teacher's difficulties are considered and visits adjusted to convenient times, with due notice given, and also if the health visitor takes an active and intelligent interest in school functions and activities.

In any community the health visitor will find she has many other pro-

fessional colleagues in allied disciplines. Two of her best known partners will be the district nurse and the midwife and she will need to meet them fairly regularly. Teaching in ante-natal classes will often be shared with the midwife, and understanding and close co-operation is essential, for both to deal with the appropriate aspects of preparation for motherhood, and for conflicting presentation of child-rearing practice to be avoided.

Co-operation with the general practitioner is of growing importance, with the modern emphasis on family care, and wholeness of the individual in relation to promotion of health. In many areas it is becoming the custom for a health visitor to become attached to a firm of general practitioners and a recognized working relationship exists. The health visitor will be concerned with the families on the register of the practice, carrying out her usual function with them, in close liaison with the doctor. In this way she can relieve the doctor of some of the more social aspects of his work, and deal with the normal aspects of child-rearing, which would be very time-consuming for the doctors during surgery hours. She is also available in her capacity as a health educator.

In this context the health visitor needs to be sure that she retains her functions and that her true potential is fully realized. This form of co-operation can achieve an ideal service for the family where it exists — where it does not, a good working relationship must be established. This is best attained if the health visitor calls on the doctor at the most convenient times, and is prepared to share her knowledge of the family background when necessary.

These then are some of the most essential colleagues with whom the health visitor needs to maintain good co-operation. There are many others, of course, including those in the health education departments, the churches and the many social workers in the various voluntary agencies, and the officials in the local government departments, but to continue the list would become tedious.

There are also some important contacts among the lay workers in her area. It is useful to know those who are on the local committees of Darby and Joan clubs, youth clubs and mother's clubs and church activities, as these groups often provide good openings for health education, or securing support in local activities.

The importance of social occasions should never be overlooked, as they often provide the opportunity for meeting in a relaxed and informal atmosphere which smooths the way for further co-operation, both with lay and professional workers. Case conferences provide a similar opportunity for staff from the various departments to share their information, and co-ordinate their activities. This can be very useful in deciding on the most efficient way of handling difficult families, with the greatest economy of time and energy and the minimum of staff.

Ultimately the same principles are basic to co-operation in all these situations. The health visitor will find her knowledge of psychology and sociology helps considerably in understanding the other person's point of view, and gives insight into her own reactions. She will have gained a useful appreciation of the importance of human motivation, of handling aggression, or insecurity, and will understand the effects of fatigue and strain and the benefits of relaxation. This all helps in tolerating differences arising from varied trainings and other disciplines. The most important factors lie in knowing the function of other members in the team; in establishing good communications; maintaining the best possible relationships between individual members by understanding, courtesy, mutual agreement. This will ensure the greatest economy and efficiency in the services offered to the family and ensure the general happiness and well-being of all members of the team.

References

1. *Porter Lee "Interviewing" in Mary Antoinette,* Cannon and Philip Klein (eds.) Social Care Work. Columbia U. Press.
2. *The First and Last Personal Freedom,* J. KRISHN'MURTI (Harper).

Suggested Reading

Essentials in Interviewing, ANN. F. FENLASON (Harper & Row).

Interviewing in the Social Services, ELIZABETH DE SCHWEINITZ and KARL DE SCHWEINITZ (National Council of Social Work).

Interviewing, its Principals and Methods, ANNETTE GARRETT (Family Welfare Association of America).

5. Home Visiting

MARION LOVELAND

Home Visiting Practice

SECTION 24(1) in Part III of the National Health Service Act, 1946, states:

> It shall be the duty of every local health authority to make provision in their area for the visiting of persons in their homes by visitors to be called "health visitors" for the purpose of giving advice as to the care of young children, persons suffering from illness, and expectant and nursing mothers and as to the measures to prevent the spread of infection.

This section of the act made the health of the whole household the concern of the health visitor. From this it will also be seen that the health visitor has a prime function; health education and social advice. More important is that she is now regarded as the long-term family visitor. She has statutory obligations to visit the homes where there are young children.

The health visitor in order to fulfil her functions as educator and adviser must have a good basis of knowledge not only of the academic kind laid down in her nursing and health visitor training, but she must also have a knowledge of the world around her and the stresses and strains to which people are subjected. She must endeavour to remain outside emotional involvement with the families she visits, whilst remaining approachable, friendly and sympathetic. She must above all be a good listener and be prepared to give her advice in a manner acceptable to her client and in terms that can be easily understood. She must be prepared to have her advice questioned and even rejected and must meet rebuffs with equanimity. The health visitor must be a person of integrity with whom confidences are safe. She must be a loyal and co-operative colleague prepared to give good service to the community she serves.

Good basic knowledge required by a health visitor is given during her special training. How to use this knowledge is the practice of health visiting.

The first thing a health visitor must do is to establish priorities in her visiting programme. The most important aspect of her work is still the care of the young child within its family. The mental, physical and environmental aspects are all important. The over-protected child needs as much care as the neglected. Other groups coming high in the list of priorities requiring supervision are the expectant mother, the incomplete family, the mentally disordered, the handicapped, the inadequate family and the elderly. She also has scope for health education with those in the middle years and she is brought more closely in contact with this group where she is attached to the general practitioner. This pattern is spreading throughout the country and the health visitor is therefore able to broaden her function. The health visitor in the school health service, and her place in health education are dealt with elsewhere, but it will be appreciated that all home visiting is health education.

A pattern of visiting has to be established as soon as possible. Much of this will depend on modes of transport and the pattern of the area. If time and energy are to be preserved, visits in adjoining streets will be planned to be done together. Before setting out, the health visitor decides which visits she wishes to do and which need to be done. Care must be taken that certain areas are not over-visited, particularly where the child population is high, to the exclusion of other areas where families are well established or the population is older. The health visitor soon learns which are good days for visiting her clients, and when they will be in.

Records of families are held by every health visitor. It is the subject of discussion whether these cards should be taken out when visiting, but most health visitors will want to have some record with them as an *aide-mémoire* when they visit the families, but it is generally accepted that record cards are not produced during the visit, as some families may resent it if they think records are kept about them, and the relationships between the families and the health visitor, which are so important to her work, might be broken.

The health visitor will tell her clients where she can be found, the times she is available for consultation and her telephone number. Where the health visitor works from an office or clinic she will be there as a rule at set times during the day. Health visitors in very rural areas who work from home must arrange set times for being available. Most health visitors have fixed appointments each week, such as infant welfare clinics, and relaxation classes, but where the health visitor is doing school work these sessions are generally fixed for her by the school medical clerk. Apart from these appointments the health visitor is free to plan her own visiting programme. No strict pattern of visiting is laid down and in some cases it may be necessary for her to visit daily at first. When she has established a relationship with a family and the members seem to be getting on all right, she will begin to lengthen the time between her visits, making sure that she can be contacted if the family wants her to visit or to make an appointment. When the health visitor makes an appointment she must endeavour to keep it punctually. Good relationships develop when the mother feels that she can rely on the health visitor to visit her when she is worried and to spend time listening to her troubles.

Before setting out to do any visits the health visitor should know the purpose of her visits. Aimless visiting serves no useful purpose.

The Expectant Mother

Visiting the expectant mother is largely educative. If it is the health visitor's first contact with the family she will have to introduce herself and explain why she has come. The health visitor may or may not know what arrangements have been made for the confinement and she must be prepared, if questioned, to state how she became informed of the pregnancy. Often the health visitor will be asked to advise about the arrangements for the confinement. The mother's wishes must be considered but in the *Report on Neonatal Mortality and Morbidity* a joint committee of the Royal College of Obstetricians and Gynaecologists and the British Paediatric Association recommended that the following should be delivered in hospital:

1. All primigravidae;
2. All women who have had four or more children;
3. All whose labours are likely to be abnormal;
4. Multiple pregnancies;
5. Where the baby is likely to be small or weak;
6. Where home conditions are unsuitable.

These recommendations must be borne in mind when advising the expectant mother. Special attention must be paid to the mother who is Rhesus negative and may develop antibodies, so that arrangements are made for the baby who may need an exchange transfusion.

Certain advantages and disadvantages are also kept in mind when discussing with the mother, the arrangements for home or hospital confinement.

The Advantages of Home Confinement

1. The mother feels happier in her own home with her family around her.

2. The mother often does not want to be separated from her other children and husband.

3. The baby is part of the family from the beginning and routine to suit the family can be established.

4. The mother will receive advice which will suit her individual needs in her own home.

The Disadvantages of Home Confinement

1. There is not constant attention for the mother and baby, and skilled help is not so readily available.
2. The mother may tend to assume her household responsibilities too soon where there is inadequate help in the home.
3. The mother's diet may be neglected.
4. The expense is greater, as domestic help has to be paid for.

Advantages of Hospital Confinement

1. There is constant medical and nursing care.
2. The mother is free from household responsibilities.
3. Hospital care is free.

Disadvantages of Hospital Confinement

1. Risk of infection to mother and baby is greater.
2. The opportunities for teaching the mother how to care for her child are less.
3. There is separation from the family.

Many hospitals notify the local health authority of bookings made. The health visitor will make sure that the mother is clear about attending for ante-natal examination and stress the importance of the mother's attendance. She will discuss preparations for the baby when it is born and will endeavour to find out how much the mother understands about the growth of the foetus, give advice on diet, exercise, clothing, rest and work during pregnancy, make sure that the mother knows how to obtain welfare milk, vitamins, and any insurance benefits due to her.

There is provision of dental care for the expectant mother and the health visitor will advise her to have her teeth inspected early on in pregnancy, in order that treatment, where necessary, can be completed before confinement.

Infant feeding will be a subject of importance to the mother and the health visitor will listen to the mother's own views on feeding and support her in her decision. She will give the mother reasons why breast feeding is advantageous both to mother and infant, leaving the mother to make up her own mind how she will feed her infant.

The health visitor must be prepared to answer questions on marital relationships during pregnancy and immediately after delivery. She must help the mother to accept changes in attitudes of the husband, and will invite her to attend any mothercraft classes which are held. If possible an evening session should be arranged so that husbands can attend. The health visitor will tell the mother where she can be found, that she is willing to help her, that she will call again and will continue visiting when the baby is born. The health visitor will pass back information she acquires to the hospital or midwife.

The Unmarried Mother

The health visitor may be the first person who is consulted by an unmarried mother. The importance of making arrangements for the confinement and for adequate ante-natal care must be stressed and the health visitor will discuss with the mother the future of the child, trying to find out what the mother's plans are. Whilst pointing out to the mother that the child needs a complete family for its full development, the health visitor must not persuade the mother to take any particular course of action she may later regret. The health visitor must ascertain the mother's financial position, telling her what statutory benefits are due to her under social security, and how they may be obtained. The health visitor should co-operate with voluntary agencies caring for the unmarried mother and their specialized workers.

The health visitor will continue to visit the unmarried mother, giving her support, advice and guidance.

If the mother returns home with her child, the health visitor will continue to visit her and keep the baby under observation, and will advise her to attend the infant welfare centre with her child.

The New Baby

The mother with the new baby, especially the first, is always very anxious. She wants to do the best for her infant physically, materially, mentally and socially. She will be subjected to pressures from relations, friends and neighbours. The health visitor must help her to sort out all the information on child care she receives from these people, as well as what she reads, hears on the wireless and sees on the television. Above all, the health visitor must support and encourage her and give the mother the full benefit of her professional knowledge.

The health visitor will want to find out certain information from the mother, particularly in regard to her general health, diet, rest and general management of the household. If it appears necessary for the mother to have some domestic help the health visitor may be able to arrange this.

The condition of the baby should be found out, especially with regard to feeding, eyes, umbilicus, skin, bowel action and sleeping arrangements.

Anxieties about feeding arise in the early weeks after delivery and these problems must be solved jointly by the mother and the health visitor. It is advantageous to all concerned that the health visitor should know the views of the mother's general practitioner about feeding; she will not want to give contradictory advice which will confuse the mother. The mother's views on infant feeding must be discussed and her wishes considered when choosing artificial feeding.

During the early months feeding is an important aspect of child health. Principles on which feeding advice will be given are that the child should thrive, be contented, sleep well and develop normally within its own limits. The health visitor will ensure that the child is receiving an adequate diet and that vitamin additives are given. She will have a plan for advising the mother on weaning. The care and sterilization of feeding bottles, teats, etc., will be discussed where there is artificial feeding.

Advice will be given about immunization programmes, and it will be pointed out that this can be carried out by the general practitioner or at the local authority clinics. The health visitor must be able to discuss with the mother why these procedures are necessary and the advisability of completing the course.

Dentition, as it occurs, will be a subject for discussion with the mother and advice given in the care of the teeth. Special facilities are available through the School Dental Service for the care of the young child's teeth.

During the course of her visiting, the health visitor will be aware of the early signs of mental stress, particularly in relation to the expectant mother and the mother with the new baby.

Health education comes into every visit, the health visitor teaching the mother by informal discussion about the dangers of infection to the new baby, the prevention of accidents in the home, the importance of keeping the baby warm and the management of her new family. She will stress the importance of her attendance at the post-natal examination.

The health visitor must inform the mother of the location and time of the infant welfare centre and where she can be found if needed. She will also tell her that she will visit again, perhaps making an appointment to suit the mother. If this is done the health visitor must keep her appointment punctually, whatever happens.

The Premature Baby

If the mother has had to return home without the baby, the health visitor will visit her to give reassurance and support, and to prepare the mother for the baby's return. She will need advice on the preparation of the sleeping arrangements for the baby and the importance of being able to maintain the room temperature to prevent cold injury. If the mother is expressing the breast milk and taking it to the hospital, the health visitor must be ready to give her help and advice and to see that a good standard of cleanliness is maintained, to prevent the spread of infection. The health of the mother must be safeguarded so that she is ready to undertake the care of the child when he returns home.

The Toddler

Visiting toddlers is as important as visiting young infants. The child is showing his independence and, with it, his ability to speak and question. The mother will need help to understand that temper tantrums, food fads and negativism are just normal phases of development and the health visitor will advise her on how to deal with these. She may need help on how to prepare the toddler for the arrival of the new baby and how to deal with his behaviour towards it. Some mothers may need help on toys for the toddler and the importance of his meeting other children of his own age. Shoes, clothing, diet will be subjects for the informal teaching during the visits.

An important aspect of child care, during the years after the child becomes mobile, is the prevention of accidents in the home. These are the years of growing independence, inquisitiveness and imitation, and the child will have to be safeguarded from poisons of all kinds, pills and fires. It is an offence to have an unguarded fire where there are young children. The health visitor must use all her persuasive powers to see that the mother protects her child against any accidents, without curbing his activities too much.

Many local health authorities hold special toddler clinics and the health visitor will invite the mother to bring the child to these sessions. At these clinics the appointment system is usual; this gives time for the toddler to be examined and for the doctor, mother and health visitor to have a leisurely talk. The toddler will usually be weighed and measured and it is advantageous if a dental surgeon is available to examine the child's teeth. There should also be close co-operation with the child guidance clinic, in case there is need to refer the mother and child for treatment where there are behaviour problems. The health visitor will try to enlist the help of voluntary workers to look after the toddlers if consultation is needed with the mother alone. Having special sessions for toddlers gives opportunity to study behaviour problems and for preventive work in this respect.

The importance of keeping up to date with immunization schedules will be pointed out. The last visit to the toddler before he starts school is important. The mother must prepare the child for this separation and she may need guidance on how to do this, as well as help with practical preparation of the child, such as tying shoes, etc.

The Handicapped

The health visitor will often be the liaison officer between the general practitioner and the patient, and the hospital and the home. With her nursing background, her experience in home visiting and knowledge of the social services, she is able to help the general practitioner in the care of handicapped people.

A handicap has social implications and has repercussions on the whole family. The health visitor can supply information on the home circumstances for the hospital, which will be of value when the patient is to be discharged. Whether the handicapped person is young or old the family will need a great deal of support. The mother faced with a handicapped child may feel guilty or reject the child; she must be helped with these feelings and the health visitor must show her that she is willing to help and advise. She must be prepared to spend time discussing the future with the mother and show her that there are many ways of helping and that there are facilities available at all stages of the child's life for education, and later for employment. She must help the mother to accept the child and with her knowledge of the normal, will be able to explain what can be expected of the child within his handicap. In order to do this the mother must be willing to take the child for assessment and be helped to see the wisdom of proposed lines of action. The health visitor can try to link the family with other families with handicapped children so that the mother can get help from those in similar circumstances. When a member of the family becomes handicapped later in life, the health visitor must be willing and able to get practical help, and give advice on aids which can be provided in the home. She will have to see that the financial circumstances are safeguarded and to tell the family where voluntary and statutory help is available.

The Blind

It is important that the health visitor should realize how necessary it is to detect blindness as early as possible. The shock to the family of a child born blind is very great, and the mother may become over-protective and do everything for the child. She must be helped to appreciate that affection and security are important but that the child must develop independence. The blind child's other senses must be given extra stimulation. He must be allowed to handle common objects and, when he begins to crawl, he must be able to explore the room. The mother should be advised about having things in the same position all the time, so that he becomes familiar with them and will soon find his way about, but he must be protected from danger from fires, knives, etc. When he begins to walk, he will find his way about by the furniture and, with help, will be able to go up and down stairs. Throughout his training the mother must help him gain experience and become independent. There will be frustrations, but gradually he will build up his self-respect. It may be necessary for the child to go into a home, and the Royal National Institute for the Blind runs homes for very young blind children. They can be sent there at any age but if the home conditions are good the child will remain with his family. But it must be remembered that special methods are required to teach the blind child which may necessitate his being away from home.

When blindness occurs later in life, adjustment to it needs guidance. The newly blind may have a home teacher or may be admitted to a residential home to re-establish confidence in daily activities. It will be necessary to provide training if the newly blind cannot continue in their previous occupation.

The Deaf

Health visitors are now prepared in the method of testing hearing in the young baby. Any child appearing to fail these tests is referred for further tests, assessment and action if there is any doubt. The mother must understand that if her child is found to be deaf, she must co-operate with specialists in auditory training. It should be explained to her that, if the child does not hear, he will not speak. Teaching should start when the child would normally be ready to listen, and continue during the second year, when he would normally be ready to speak. Young deaf children can be supplied with a hearing aid and the mother must be instructed in the importance of wearing it. Hearing aids are loaned free under the National Health Service and batteries are provided free. The partially deaf are more difficult to detect and every child who appears to be slow to talk or has a speech defect or behaviour problems should be tested to find out if the hearing is normal: many children thought to be subnormal have been found to have a hearing defect.

Tuberculosis

The health visitor may have the care of tuberculous patients in the course of her duties. She will be the liaison between the chest physician and the patient. Many patients will wonder why the health visitor comes and the purpose of her visit must always be made clear. The health visitor will make sure that the patient understands the doctor's instructions and is carrying them out, particularly in regard to his own regimen and to prevent the spread of infection. She will have to spend time tracing contacts of the infected person and advise them to attend for examination, and she will ascertain that the family is having help where there are economic problems. Where the husband or wife is affected with tuberculosis, she may be asked about pregnancy and marital relationships. She must be prepared to advise them to seek further help from the Family Planning Association which may be willing to send a visitor to the family at home. The health visitor may be asked by the hospital to provide a report on the home conditions of a patient ready for discharge, and this can be of great help to the staff of the hospital. She will keep in touch with the family whilst the patient is in hospital, stressing importance of a follow-up examination of the family, and preparing them for the patient's return home. The health visitor will know of the schemes of rehabilitation and after-care of the patient who has suffered from tuberculosis and will be able to explain them to the family and stress the advisability of accepting any recommendations made. In some areas specialist health visitors are employed whose responsibility is the care of those suffering from tuberculosis and other chest diseases.

Mental Disorder

Mental subnormality causes great family stress. There will be guilt feelings between the parents, each subconsciously blaming the other. The health visitor must be prepared for this and must listen to what may be said as reasons for the subnormality, knowing all the time that neither parent is to blame; she must try and explain this to the family. The repercussions on other members of the family may be very severe and, whilst realizing that the best place for a mentally subnormal child is a good home, it may be in the family's best interest for the child to be admitted for long-term care. This does not alleviate the feelings of guilt and can on occasions make family relationships more difficult. The family will need a great deal of help, advice and support, and the health visitor must accept this and must give time to these families.

With her knowledge of normal child development, she will help the family to accept the slow progress the child makes, and will help them to realize that patience and love are needed to deal with the child. Just as ordinary children need some discipline, so will the mentally subnormal child, but again he will be slower to learn the *mores* of behaviour which are expected of him.

As with any handicapped child, assessment is important, and the health visitor will advise the parent to take the child for physical and intelligence assessments, and to prepare the family to accept the advice given. She must help the mother to train the child in good habits, making him socially acceptable and able to lead as normal a life as possible. The health visitor must be sure that the physical and social health of the child is safeguarded and that good standards of hygiene are maintained. It is now possible for the severely subnormal to attend a training centre, and it is important that the mother co-operates with the staff of the training centre in everything they are trying to do to help the child.

The health visitor can often be the go-between with neighbours and acquaintances, and may often enlist help. She may also persuade the parents to join the local branch of the National Society for Mentally Handicapped Children or, if there is no branch, suggest they start one, so that parents in similar circumstances can meet together and share their problems. It is sometimes possible for the child to be taken into a special hospital for a short period, so that the family may have a rest. The questions of education and employment will be a source of worry to the family and the health visitor will be able to inform the parents of arrangements which can be made for the child.

Some health visitors, who have attended training courses at psychiatric hospitals, are now undertaking home visiting of families where there has been mental illness. Some of these health visitors are attached to the psychiatric hospitals and work in co-operation with the staff.

Mental welfare officers are employed by local authorities and the health visitors will have close liaison with them in cases of mental disorder in adults.

The Elderly

The health visitor's duties have extended to include the needs of the elderly, whether living within the family or alone.

There is no system of registering the elderly, and the health visitor will find them in a variety of ways. When she pays her first visit she will have to assess the situation and decide what needs the most urgent attention. Having decided, she will contact the relevant person giving all particulars. She can help the family to adjust to meet the needs of the elderly and can encourage the old person living alone to use the statutory and voluntary resources available. The health visitor will work in close co-operation with the general practitioner, district nurse, and geriatric workers, in obtaining the best for the old person. She may be able to arrange for the infirm old person, living within the family, to go into temporary accommodation to enable the family to have a rest or go on holiday. She may have opportunities of promoting neighbourliness, and linking those who want to help with those who need help.

In visiting the elderly, the health visitor must be aware of the potential dangers causing home accidents. By constant supervision, failing health can be seen, and action taken before it is too late. The main problems of the elderly are increasing feebleness, due to degeneration of all systems, loneliness and unsuitable housing. As long as possible old people must be helped to keep their independence. They like to remain in their own homes with their familiar possessions around them, and the health visitor must obtain help from voluntary and statutory organizations to preserve this.

It is most important in the visiting of the elderly to ensure that promises and appointments are kept. The elderly enjoy visitors and like to think that people are interested in them.

Having discussed in detail certain handicapped persons the health visitor may have to deal with, it must be stressed that children who are on the "at risk" register will need special attention. They will have to be watched carefully during the early years and, at any sign of abnormality, assessment examinations may be necessary.

The health visitor must be aware, when dealing with handicapped persons, of the facilities available to them through the Ministry of Labour, Ministry of Social Security and the numerous voluntary agencies, and there should be close co-operation between the health visitor and the welfare department.

The handicapped must be encouraged to join in any local organizations available to them. Children should be allowed to take part in any activities so that they can attain a sense of achievement and independence.

The health visitor must recognize the importance of promotion of mental health, particularly with the families with young children for it is in this aspect that real preventive work lies.

The Abnormal Family

The Ministry of Health issued a circular (*Health of Children. Prevention of Break Up of Families* 27/54) in which concern was expressed at the bad effects on the mental health of children, following the break up of families. It also pointed out that the prevention of physical and mental ill health was the special care of the local health authority.

There are different types of abnormal families, among them the incomplete family, the broken family and the family with a multiplicity of problems.

The health visitor's function in dealing with such families is to assess the problems and needs and to take appropriate action. During the course of home visiting she is particularly well placed in recognizing the early signs of family failure. She is able to offer advice and help which may enable the family to overcome their difficulties. She is in such a position that other workers will contact her when any signs of difficulty are seen; these workers may be the school welfare officer, the housing manager where there is rent defaulting, the home nurse, etc.

The work with abnormal families is very time-consuming, but it is a very important part of her work. The health visitor must know to whom she can go when more intensive work is needed.

Many local authorities have set up co-ordinating committees and have designated officers, whose duty is to co-ordinate the work of the many voluntary and statutory agencies concerned with difficult families. These officers will also call a meeting of the workers involved, in order to try to decide the best way to deal with them. The health visitor is present at these meetings and will bring to them information obtained during home visits, which will be of great value in helping to make decisions. Where there are children under 5 years of age, she has a statutory obligation to visit to keep an eye on the children's progress. Health education can be of little value where there are many problems and the health visitor must make every attempt to remove or alleviate the problems in order that her advice can be used, but above all she must give continued support to the family, whoever undertakes intensive care.

The Nurseries and Child Minders Act, 1948

Under this Act local health authorities have a duty to keep registers and to inspect:

1. Premises where children are looked after for the day or the substantial part of the day, for a period not exceeding 6 days;
2. Persons who receive children under the age of 5, to be looked after for the day or for a substantial part of the day, for a period not exceeding 6 days, for reward.

In some areas health visitors are required to make the assessment visit when persons apply to start a day nursery and, more usually, when a person has applied to be a registered daily minder.

In the case of the daily minder it is "the person" who is registered and the health visitor must be sure that the applicant is a suitable person, that she has an understanding of small children and that she has suitable premises in which to care for them. Following registration the health visitor will visit the daily minder to ensure the welfare of the children and to give advice on their care, particularly in regard to feeding, the prevention of accidents, and the prevention of the spread of infection.

When approached by any person wishing to become a daily minder, the health visitor will advise the inquirer to apply for registration. A daily minder must apply if she is not a relative of the children and if she receives more than two children coming from more than one household; she may apply in other circumstances, for example when she minds only one child, and the health visitor should point out the advisability of voluntary registration.

When the health visitor is required to visit a registered day nursery, she will make sure that the number of children does not exceed the number allowed in the registration; that the welfare of the children is safeguarded and that adequate records are kept and are available for inspection. She has an important duty to prevent the spread of infection and local authorities have powers to require that no child is received if he appears to be suffering from any infectious disease or, in the case of a daily minder, that no child shall be received where any member of the household is suffering from any infectious disease specified by the local authority.

The local authority has a duty to inspect day nurseries and child minders at any reasonable time, and will appoint an authorized person to do the inspection. There is machinery for the inspector to be issued with an authenticated document if admission is refused. Where the authorized person is the health visitor, she knows the majority of families in her district and the relationships are such that the use of statutory powers is usually unnecessary but these are provided as a safeguard in times of emergency. There are some loopholes in this Act, as there is divergence of interpretation as to the meaning of "a substantial part". Some day nurseries and daily minders take children for a morning or an afternoon only and therefore do not come under the Act; in some cases these arrangements are very unsatisfactory.

It is important that the health visitor visits regularly all children in day nurseries and with daily minders. Her training particularly prepares her for observation and assessment necessary for the proper care of children, notably of the emotional, physical, social and developmental needs, and she is the person to undertake these visits.

Recommended Reading

The Psychological Development of the Child, PAUL H. MUSSEN (Prentice Hall).
The Developmental Progress of Infants and Young Children, MARY D. SHERIDAN, M.A., M.D., D.C.H. (H.M.S.O.).
Infant Feeding, ALAN MONCRIEFF (Edward Arnold).
Report of the Sub-Committee on the Prevention of Prematurity and the Care of Premature Infants (H.M.S.O.).
Change of Life. Facts and Fallacies of Middle Age, Joan Malleson (Penguin).
The Psychology of Human Ageing, D.B. Bromley (Pelican).

6. The Health Visitor in the Health Centres

Marion Loveland

The Health Visitor and the Welfare Centre

IN ORDER to understand the functions and role of the health visitor in the welfare centre today, it is necessary to look at the history of the Maternity and Child Welfare Movement.

In 1892 Dr. Pierre Bandin, Professor of Clinical Obstetrics in the University of Paris, established the first infant consultation clinic in the Charité Hospital in Paris. He encouraged the mothers to bring their babies each week to his clinic during the first 2 years of life. In order to continue satisfactory breast feeding, he paid special attention to the health of the mothers. At every visit the infant's weight was recorded together with a report on the child's general progress. When it was necessary to wean the infant, sterilized milk was supplied to the mothers, thus reducing the incidence of contamination. Infant consultation clinics spread rapidly in France and the provision of sterilized milk played an important part.

In 1899 the St. Helen's milk depot was started, and many other towns soon followed. In some of the milk depots the infants were weighed, and those children who received the milk were kept under supervision by health visitors.

In 1905 the first international congress on infant welfare was held in Paris and was followed in 1906 by the first national conference. This conference gave a powerful impetus to the infant welfare movement. "Maternity and Child Welfare Centres", municipal and voluntary, increased rapidly, largely due to the influence of Dr. Eric Pritchard who established a voluntary centre in 1906 in St. Marylebone. The advice given in this clinic was practical and aimed at keeping the infants well, rather than treating them when ill. There the mothers were interviewed individually and given advice to meet their own needs. At this time the most important part of the work was weighing the baby, but this met with resistance on the part of some mothers, who thought it brought bad luck.

Soon after its establishment the centre started group teaching, and this led to the opening of the St. Pancras School for Mothers in 1907. As well as infant management, taught in the Schools for Mothers, there were classes in sewing, cooking and general household management. Even then it was realized that benefit could be obtained from the stimulation of interest within a group, but it was questioned whether this was as useful as the individual consultation. Even today the personal interview in the home is of greater value to the mother, although she gains a great deal if she attends mothercraft groups and chats to others in similar circumstances. Even in these early days the work at the centre was augmented by the visits to the home of the health visitor, who ensured that the advice of the doctor was carried out.

From the beginning free milk was part of the service of milk depots, but in about 1907 dried milk was given. In Paris nursing mothers had been given free or cheap meals and Mrs Gordon started this service in Chelsea, opening a small restaurant for them. This idea grew and many centres started as a place where meals were provided. The provision of dried milk grew and is part of the service of many centres today.

At first the centres were mostly concerned with the care of the child in the first year of life, but gradually it was realized that the service should extend to children in the first 5 years. It also appeared that much could be done if the mother's health was attended to, and gradually the centres, which had been started for infant care, became "maternity and child welfare centres".

All through the growth of the centre movement, sick children were not treated and, if they needed treatment, they were referred to the doctor or the hospital.

Dental clinics for mothers and sunlight treatment clinics for children suffering from malnutrition were provided, but the main object of the centres was educational.

Many local authorities provided special buildings for centres and, under the 1946 National Health Service Act, health centres were to be provided.

Today the function of the welfare centre is still to help the mother to rear a healthy child. Health includes emotional as well as physical well-being, and every aspect of child care is covered in the advice given in the centre.

The Child Welfare Centre

In busy units the usual staff consists of doctor, health visitor, clinical assistant, clerk and voluntary helpers. In some country areas there may only be doctor, health visitor and voluntary helpers.

Sessions are held regularly each week or fortnight and the prime functions of the child welfare centre are the observation of normal development, health guidance and referral if there is deviation from the normal. Mothers bring their children under 5 years of age for guidance and advice. It is preferable that the centre should be within easy reach of the mothers it serves, and that the health visitor responsible for the home visiting in the area should be in attendance at the centre. This provides a continuity of advice, with advantages to both mother and health visitor. The health visitor knows the home circumstances of the family and will be able to give advice to suit their needs.

The doctor is available for specialist consultation, advice, and for giving a periodic full examination. The health visitor will give health advice and guidance. The clinic assistant and the clerk can carry out functions not requiring the specialist knowledge of the health visitor. The clinic assistant can be responsible for weighing, laying out and clearing away of clinics, the maintenance of stock and equipment; she can be in attendance with the doctor for prophylactic sessions when these are held separately from the child welfare sessions. The clerical assistant is necessary in a busy centre to deal with appointments, telephone calls, the statistical returns supplied by the health visitors, and the sale and stocks of nutrients sold in the centre.

There is still an important place for voluntary workers in the centres, such as supervising toddlers whilst the mothers are otherwise engaged, making tea, etc.

In some areas an experienced health visitor is responsible for the administration of the welfare centre. She has to see that the whole centre runs smoothly and has to arrange the sessions which take place. She may also be responsible for the replacement of stock and equipment and the supervision of the cleanliness of the premises. Where she holds the position of centre superintendent, she may have to act in an advisory capacity to other health visitors based at the centre. She also has to arrange for relief during holidays, vacancies and sickness, and for the reception of visitors. The responsibility for the programmes for student health visitors now lies with the field-work instructors, but the centre superintendent may have to arrange programmes for other students. She will also be responsible for the care of any drugs kept in the centre.

In some areas a health visitor may have to go out with the mobile health unit, visiting areas where no static centre is available. She will hold an infant welfare centre in the unit and often immunization procedures are undertaken. It is the health visitor's responsibility to see that everything required for the session is in the unit, and that it is left ready for the next session on return to base.

In smaller units and mobile centres it may be possible for the health visitor to manage with a voluntary worker only, who deals with the sale of nutrients and the clerical work. At no time should the health visitor be expected to sell nutrients and only in the small units should she be responsible for stocks and finances of these nutrients.

If possible a separate room should be available if the health visitor wants to have a private consultation with a mother, but being in the room where mothers are handling their children and listening to their talk she will gain a lot of information, and if she feels a mother needs more advice she can see her privately or arrange to visit her at home. The mother may have come for the sole purpose of seeing the health visitor and she must have the privacy which is desirable.

The routine of a child welfare centre follows a fairly common pattern. The mother attending for the first time is met by the health visitor and taken to a table where she is required to register. She is then handed an attendance card which may or may not have space for the child's weight to be recorded. Babies attending for the first time are generally weighed, and unless there is any real contra-indication the child should be weighed naked. The health visitor should if possible see the child being weighed, so that she can observe the child whilst it is undressed. She will also be able to observe the mother's handling of the child. Usually the child is seen by the medical officer at the first attendance and the health visitor can give the doctor much valuable information about the home and family circumstances. This should be an unhurried consultation and, if the child continues to make satisfactory progress, it will not be necessary for the doctor to see it at every attendance.

At subsequent visits, apart from periodic full examinations, the child will be weighed if the mother so wishes and she will have a health consultation with the health visitor, who may consider it necessary to refer the mother to the doctor for further consultation. On the other hand, the mother may request such a consultation. To many mothers weight is an understandable sign of the child's progress and the child should be weighed whenever the mother desires it, but she should be led to understand that this is not the only indication of a child's progress and there are many other factors which must be taken into consideration. The health visitor may consider it necessary to follow up a centre attendance with a home visit.

At some welfare centres demonstrations or talks are given by health visitors or invited specialist speakers but group health education sessions should be arranged on days other than the child welfare sessions. The health visitor would have to make arrangements for adequate supervision of babies and toddlers at the centre.

If child welfare sessions are held in church halls or huts hired for the purpose, the health visitor will be responsible for seeing that adequate preparations are made for the session and that the rooms are cleared up afterwards. Sometimes the health visitor will be asked to start a child welfare centre in hired premises to meet the needs of local mothers. She must then take stock of the accommodation available and use it to the best advantage. Ideally there should be a waiting room which can also be used for serving cups of tea, displays, the sale of nutrients and the table at which the mothers can register their attendance. There should be a room where the infants can be weighed, a health visitor's consultation room, and a doctor's consultation room. There should also be some lavatory accommodation and a place for the mothers to leave their perambulators. Suitable furniture, if possible, should be provided and there should be baskets or bowls in which mothers can place the child's clothes if he has to be undressed. The hall should be kept clean and warm, and arrangements must be made for this with the owners of the premises.

At child welfare centres immunization is carried out. The health visitor must encourage the mothers to make use of this service if they do not intend to go to their general practitioner.

Special sessions for toddlers are held in some areas and the health visitor can supply the doctor with important information obtained in the course of home visiting. Mothers and children come to toddlers' clinics by invitation and there is a full medical examination at each visit. Behaviour and development can be studied and the toddler is weighed. Time must be available for the mother to discuss problems with the doctor or health visitor and for guidance to be given. If possible a dentist should be available, so that dental advice can be given.

Health Centres

Health centres, as envisaged in the National Health Service Act, 1946, were to be buildings where general practitioners, dentists, pathologists and specialists, together with local health authority services, were to be housed in one place. Because of financial restrictions, some local authorities have not been able to build health centres to any great extent, but they are increasing in number at the present time. Health education is undertaken at such health centres, in addition to the other services.

Health visitors, school nurses, district nurses, midwives and social workers are provided with office accommodation and consultation rooms. There is also a large room for health education programmes.

The health visitors are responsible for running their own infant welfare centres and arranging their own health education programmes, in co-operation with their colleagues.

The Ante-natal Clinic

Much of the success of the ante-natal clinic depends on the co-operation of the midwife and health visitor. The guiding principle must be the health and welfare of the mother, and all the staff will help her to realize that pregnancy is a normal function and that they are there to help her maintain good health during her pregnancy. The health visitor will be responsible for the administration of the clinic and for the health education programme. She will see that specimens for blood tests are obtained and despatched, and will pass on information to the hospital or midwife responsible for the confinement. In many areas, those mothers who are having a home confinement attend the general practitioner – obstetrician's clinic, where the domiciliary midwife is in attendance, but local authority relaxation and mothercraft classes are available to them. The health visitor will often be responsible for organizing these classes and will arrange the programme. She will enlist the help of midwives in some of the sessions and, if she does not teach the relaxation exercises herself, may have the help of a physiotherapist. The aim of these classes is to help the mother to arrive at her confinement with confidence, free from undue stress, with some knowledge of the physiology of labour and prepared to accept her new responsibilities when the baby is born.

Relaxation and Mothercraft Clinics

The demand for these clinics has increased tremendously during the past few years. For a long time health visitors have given talks to expectant mothers on a variety of subjects. As a rule the health visitor who is responsible for these clinics discusses the plan and subjects with the mothers and the discussion method is of greater advantage than the formal talk. Generally, a definite time is set aside for relaxation and exercises, which the health visitor herself may conduct. Expectant mothers are very anxious for guidance and particularly receptive to education.

The health visitor will see that there is suitable equipment available for these classes and may enlist the help of a voluntary worker to make tea for the mothers attending, although sometimes this is undertaken by the mothers themselves. If the mothers request a talk from any outside specialist, the health visitor will be available to give information and addresses, or she may herself make the approach to the lecturer. Films and film strips should be available if the mothers want them, and the local midwife may be very pleased to take part in the discussions.

The importance of teaching mental health and family relationships is realized, and the health visitor will arrange classes for parents which, if held in the evenings, enable the fathers to be present.

Whichever kind of group meetings are held, the health visitor will be the person responsible for the organization and will be one of the qualified specialists available. No health education can be effective if there are barriers, and the health visitor in her contact with families, whether at home or in the clinics, must reduce these barriers, either by her own efforts or by seeking the help of other workers.

Parents' Clubs

Where these clubs are organized in connection with the welfare clinics, evening sessions are usual. Social as well as educational activities are arranged, generally by a committee of parents, but the health visitor is usually consulted about the educational programme. She may be asked to take part in the programme and has a good opportunity for her health teaching.

Sometimes social gatherings are arranged by the committees of parents' clubs and these should be encouraged by the health visitor.

Special Clinics

Some local authorities have started special clinics for asthma, diabetes, obesity, eneuresis, etc. The health visitor can provide a good deal of information on the social and environmental aspects of the child and its family which will be of use to the specialist in charge of the clinic. In return she should expect to be informed of any treatment or advice given, in order that she can interpret it to the family and reinforce the recommendations made.

It must be remembered that whatever centres or clinics the health visitor may attend, the most important aspect of her work remains the giving of health guidance and social advice in the homes of the families she visits.

7. The Work of the School Health Visitor

GRACE OWEN

WHEN we wish to understand the structure of any one of our social services in its present setting, it is always enlightening to look into the past, and see how the changing needs of the community have been met as the service has been established over the years.

Thus, in considering the role and function of the school health visitor in the School Health Service, it is interesting to examine its origins, to gain an understanding of the situation as we find it today.

The function of the school health visitor has changed in response to the changing needs of the school child, and the improvements in health over the last century. It was not until 1870 that education became compulsory for all children in this country, and before this date there was no way of bringing all children together for a general appraisal of their physical condition.

Early in the nineteenth century the only provision for education, other than for the very wealthy, had been in the small schools run by certain religious organizations, or the "ragged schools". Many children worked long hours in the factories and mines, and in 1838 Lord Shaftesbury drew attention to the state of their health, observing that he found children so deformed that they appeared as "all shapes of the letters of the alphabet".

Conditions improved a little during the next few decades, as Factory Acts were passed and public conscience aroused, but with the advent of compulsory education in 1870 it was realized that many children were unable to benefit owing to poor health and malnutrition and many were discovered to be ill-clad and verminous.

It was not until 20 years later, however, in 1890, that any real progress was made, when the first school medical officer was appointed in London, and 2 years later the first school nurse. In 1895 the London School Nurses' Society was formed with five nurses who worked on a voluntary basis, and in 1904 the London County Council established its own School Nursing Service. Most of the work done by the nurses in these organizations, however, was with handicapped children.

At the beginning of the twentieth century, several events occurred which attracted attention to the appalling health of the young people of this country. The examination of recruits for the Boer War revealed many physical defects, 40–60 per cent of the men being unfit to serve. In 1903 the Royal Commission on Physical Training in Scotland found much evidence of physical disability and ill-health, among school children. The Inter-departmental Committee on Physical Deterioration of 1904 was appointed to investigate these allegations and suggest means to deal with the situation, and their research endorsed the facts already known. Other surveys, such as Rowntree's Study on Poverty in York, also emphasized the need of the school child.

The first attempt to provide relief in a practical way came in the form of the Education (Provision of Meals) Act of 1906, which gave local education authorities power to provide meals for children in elementary schools, when they were unable to gain from their education, owing to malnutrition. This was followed in 1907 by the Education (Administrative Provisions) Act which made it the duty of local education authorities to provide for the medical examination of children attending elementary schools, and also to make the necessary arrangements for treatment required, thus necessitating the appointment of school nurses to carry out this treatment.

Facilities, however, remained limited until after World War I when it was again noticed that many recruits were still unfit. Local authorities were encouraged to develop within their powers the minor ailment and treatment clinics, and facilities were also extended to children in secondary schools. With this expansion the numbers of school nurses grew as the work of the School Medical Service became established. During the succeeding years the nature of the work began to change until in 1944 with the Education Act and the establishment of the School Health Service it became less concerned with treatment, and more with preventive measures and promotion of health.

A glance at some of the statistics available over the first half of this century will illustrate very effectively just how the situation has changed with the changing needs of the school child. In 1907, 1255 children under the age of 15 years died of rickets, and now it is a rare disease. The same year 2166 died from rheumatic fever, and in 1957 only 66. Between 1901–1910, 271 of every million children under 15 years died of scarlet fever, and 571 of every million died of diphtheria, while in 1957 there were no deaths from either disease.[1]

In the early twentieth century the incidence of children found with infested heads varied from area to area. In Liverpool it was 80 per cent and in Wimbledon 20 per cent. Today the figure from the whole country averages less than 3 per cent. In recent years changes have continued to occur. There has been a 71 per cent decrease in respiratory tuberculosis between 1953 and 1963 among school children, and the incidence of poliomyelitis was lower in 1962 and 1963 than in any other year since 1918.

Common defects found today are visual defects, dental caries, skin defects and foot defects, all minor ones if compared with those of the early 1900's. In 1963, 99·46 per cent of all children were classed as satisfactory on examination in school. Many other figures of interest illustrating these changes can be found in the Reports on the Health of the School Child over the years, but these examples will indicate the nature of the changing needs which dominate the changing nature of the school nurse's work, from treatment of defects to preventive measures and promoting health through education.

With the 1944 Education Act a new era began, the work of the School Health Service being set out in the School Health Service (Handicapped Pupils) Regulations of 1945, and subsequently in 1953 and 1959. This legislation made it the duty of local authorities to employ school nurses who should be qualified health visitors, as the numbers available increased. The function of the school health visitor in our present-day service arises out of this legislation, but it must be noted that in practice her work varies considerably according to the policy of the authority for which she works, the needs of the area and the staff available.

According to the 1964 report on the *Health of the School Child*,[1] most nurses in the School Health Service also work in other branches of the local authority services. At the end of 1962, 7449 were employed of whom 5749 had the health visitors' certificate. A Ministry of Health Circular,[2] issued in 1965 to all major local authorities, emphasized the need to consider the increasing use of ancillary staff. It was suggested that this practice should not in any way lessen the efficiency of the public health team, but would allow for fullest use to be made of the skills of qualified nurses and health visitors.

The health visitor should lead the nursing team in the School Health Service, supported by, state registered and state enrolled nurses, also lay assistants. She could, with advantage, be present at the child's first medical inspection at school entry, but thereafter delegate the routine work, simply being available for consultation with the doctor at regular intervals. She would, however, need to retain full responsibility for health education and much of the home visiting. Many other routine duties in school work and clinics are suggested as being suitable for delegation to appropriate assistants. Many authorities are in fact adopting this practice and as we now go on to discuss the duties of the school health visitor, arising from her statutory function in the School Health Service, we need to remember that much of the work will often be carried out very adequately by ancillary staff.

The Duties of the School Nurse

Medical Inspections

Much of the health visitor's work in connection with school medical examinations is of a preparatory nature, and involves consultation with the school medical officer. Statutory provision is made under the 1944 Education Act for each child to be examined three times during his school life, at entrance, about the age of 11 and again on leaving. Many schools since 1953 are experimenting with other schemes, retaining only the entrance examination in full and substituting questionnaires and health assessments at other ages.[1]

Whichever scheme is used, it is common practice when the date of the examination has been arranged for the health visitor to be notified by the local education authority. A list of names of the children to receive routine examinations will be sent to the school, and additional names may be forwarded by the teachers, parents or health visitor. The parents of all children to be examined are notified—usually by the school clerical staff, and asked to return their signature agreeing to the examination and stating whether or not they expect to be present. Often additional information may be requested, concerning infectious illness, or immunization received, and the health visitor will enter this on the child's medical record card. It must be remembered that information on these medical record cards is of a confidential nature, therefore only those people directly concerned with the examination should have access to the cards.

In some areas other forms of preparation are carried out—weighing and measuring the children is rare these days, except where it is necessary for medical reasons, but screening tests for hearing and vision are usually done prior to any medical examination, and results are recorded on the medical record card. These are routine tasks which the health visitor can often delegate where assistance is available. The principle is one of selection and referral of any child where tests show deviation from the normal, or where any change in the child's behaviour or health has been noted, by teacher or health visitor.

It is necessary to co-operate with the school staff to ensure that adequate facilities are available for the doctor, and for the parents who are waiting. If there is no medical room available, alternative provision should include adequate warmth, light and washing facilities in a room where privacy and quietness are possible. Arrangements are made to ensure the children are available on time, and that appointments are kept as far as is possible.

Where the health visitor is present at the examination, her chief role is that of liaison with the doctor—of sharing any knowledge she has concerning the child's home circumstances and being prepared to convey any message from the doctor when parents are absent. She will often need to reassure anxious parents and explain any treatment necessary and ensure that instructions are understood. There are opportunities for individual health education of both parent and child. Where assistance is available and the health visitor need not remain in attendance it is important for her to arrange to be available for consultation at certain times during the examination. Follow-up visits may also be necessary in certain cases to investigate home conditions, or for explanation concerning any treatment suggested.

Cleanliness Inspections

The nature of these inspections has changed considerably over the last few years, according to the needs of the area and the policy of the local authority.

In 1947 about 8 per cent of school children were found to have infested heads, and in 1957 4 per cent, while in 1963 the number had fallen to less than 3 per cent[1]—the lowest ever. In many areas there are schools which have not had a child with a verminous head for years and routine cleanliness inspections have been abandoned. In other areas the problem still necessitates routine inspection in some schools. In any case the opportunity is generally utilized to incorporate a much more general assessment of health and personal appearance, providing individual health education for those who need it. In these circumstances it may now be known as the health assessment or hygiene survey. The frequency of the inspection also varies according to need, from a termly to an annual inspection.

It is important to make an appointment at a time convenient to the school staff, wherever possible avoiding interruption of special lessons or disruption of the school programme. Also if a school medical examination is fixed for a particular date, it is helpful to complete this general assessment of the children first, as some may need to be referred to the school doctor.

If no medical room is available, a suitable room with adequate light and privacy is essential. Older children need to be examined individually to avoid embarrassment but often the youngest children in the infants' school can be seen in small groups as they have little self-consciousness and incidental teaching can be given.

The procedure varies according to the type of assessment to be carried out, and also the staff available. This may be one of the routine jobs delegated to an assistant, as it can be a very time-consuming task.

Assuming that a full assessment of the child's condition is to be made, it is usual to start by making a general note of the child's appearance and posture, making observations when clothing is inadequate or general cleanliness not satisfactory.

In addition to inspection for infestation of the head, the general state of the hair and scalp should be noted, and there is opportunity to detect other defects such as discharging ears or eyes, visual defects, sore throats or dental caries, and refer children needing treatment to special clinics. The skin should be clean and clear from infections such as impetigo.

Hands can be examined for general cleanliness, freedom from infections, conditions such as warts, and any excessive nail biting noted. This is a very common condition at certain ages and at times of stress in school or family life, and there may be opportunities to alleviate the tension in some cases. Skin infections such as ringworm and scabies are now comparatively rare but nevertheless do occur at times.

Where the feet are examined, and this is now a common practice — plantar warts and athletes' foot are frequent infections, and the health visitor may also be on the watch for signs of flat feet, and unsuitable footwear.

Generally speaking an inspection of this kind, if properly carried out, provides an opportunity to detect any minor defect which has appeared recently, to assess the child's general progress or note any marked change of appearance or personality, and to give individual teaching as the need arises, also to follow up any serious problems detected, with a home visit or referral to the appropriate department. Consultation with the teacher will be valuable and of mutual benefit in many cases where difficulties arise, but the health visitor will need to use her discretion as to how much information she can usefully pass on without breaking confidence.

Where infested heads are found, powers of exclusion can be used if no other methods of persuasion are effective. It is often usual, especially for new offenders, for the health visitor to visit the home and offer advice and encouragement where needed, on the appropriate treatment. before resorting to the official machinery available, through the local authority for compulsory cleansing.

The value of this type of inspection or assessment depends a great deal upon the time and methodical work put into it. Many routine practices are under review, and a new pattern of assessment is emerging in many areas, more in keeping with present-day needs.

Prevention of Infection

This is another sphere of the school health visitor's work which has changed considerably over recent years. Her primary concern now is to ensure that prophylactic measures available are fully utilized by school children and a high level of immunity is maintained in all schools in her area. She may have specific duties in sessions arranged for immunization or BCG vaccination, but more often lay assistants are available for the routine work. The health visitor's responsibility lies in encouraging parents to take advantage of facilities offered. With the increased protection against the commoner infections in recent years, the health visitor's work in this field has lessened, but she may still be called upon from time to time to trace contacts or visit the homes or school in connection with infectious illness and to give advice on exclusion. Vigilance cannot be relaxed in any way and she still has the responsibility of teaching preventive measures especially in relation to general hygiene and food care as outbreaks of dysentery and food poisoning are common. Another growing problem today is that of venereal disease, and this calls for a special kind of teaching among the older children.

Home Visiting

A certain amount of time will be taken for follow-up visits as already described following school medical or cleanliness inspections. There will also be after-care visits for children who have been discharged from hospital or convalescent homes. It is important that these visits should be made promptly as the difficulties arising will often emerge during the first few days after discharge from hospital.

Where the health visitor has a school for handicapped or educationally subnormal children in her area, more home visiting may be required, as the parents of these children will need extra guidance and encouragement and it is essential to gain the fullest co-operation between the school and home, to ensure the child makes the most of his limited abilities, physically or mentally while he is at school.

Co-operation and Co-ordination

One of the most important contributions the health visitor can make to the efficiency and the smooth organization of the School Health Service is to establish good co-operation on all occasions when the medical or health teams enter the school. There are many interruptions in the teacher's programme, and if this is understood and respected there will be better co-ordination all round.

The health visitor may also find herself invited to special school functions, and it is useful to take advantage of some of these invitations. This provides an opportunity to see children and parents together, also the parents notice the health visitor taking an active interest in school activities and appreciate her co-operation with the teachers in the children's interests.

She may well be invited to join with the parent–teacher's association on various occasions. Any form of intelligent interest in the school activities will help to establish respect and mutual co-operation.

One of the difficulties increasingly evident in recent years is that children travel further to school now, and thus the health visitor will often find herself responsible for school children who are resident outside the area she normally covers. This calls for closer co-operation and mutual agreement with her colleagues concerning any home visiting needed, and also adequate communication, to ensure that the child gets the maximum benefit from the School Health Service.

Health Education

The role of the health visitor in school health education is a somewhat controversial topic, on which opinions differ widely. She is, by the very nature of her work, a health educator, and well equipped through her training and experience, with many of the skills necessary for school health education. Many would argue, however, that this is really the teacher's prerogative, and would occupy far too much of the health visitor's time, causing her work in other spheres to be neglected.

Our primary task here, however, is to discuss what, in principle, the health visitor *can* do given the opportunities, and how she can best use her skills to the greater advantage in the situation she finds in her own area. The special methods and techniques necessary for school health education will be discussed in another chapter in some detail. For the moment we are simply concerned with her role in the schools, especially in relation to all the other various demands on her area which must receive priority. It is also helpful to look at it from the point of view of the child and how his needs can best be met in this sphere.

The situation as we find it in our schools today varies considerably. The 1964 Cohen Report on Health Education[3] comments on these variations, noting the general lack of organized health education in schools and the differences found in the extent to which health and education authorities co-operate. Even when co-operation is good, only a minority of children are reached effectively. Health education is not universally a compulsory subject for teachers in training, apart from the London colleges.

In some cases there is no methodical health education, or simply isolated attempts to give "sex" education or a series of talks for leavers. In a few authorities[5] a comprehensive scheme exists for all schools in the area, organized from the health education department and the health visitor may well be an active member of the team. Some of these authorities attempt to establish the policy of the Ministry of Education (as it was in 1958) in the pamphlet issued on *Health Education*.[4] They suggest that

> ... health education is not so much a teaching subject as a form of education, pervading the whole work and life of the school, involving the headmaster and headmistress and all their staff. Every teacher has a contribution to make. ...

The Newsom Report also recommended a planned system of health education, but integrated with the school curriculum. Many experts feel that such incidental teaching, by teachers through the existing curriculum in subjects such as biology, domestic science or physical education, is likely to be vague, and should be supplemented with specific teaching in certain subjects by specialists. It is here that members of staff of the health department may be called in, and they may also act in an advisory capacity in assisting teachers in planning programmes for health teaching.

Whatever method is used it is essential that each individual child shall be educated for living—he must have opportunity to discover how his body functions, and how to adjust to the changing environment, and to acquire attitudes which will lead him towards being a responsible member of the community, having a well-integrated personality. He needs both factual knowledge and an understanding of the principles of application. These are just a few of the current trends of thought in the field of school health education, and it is with this situation in mind that the health visitor needs to formulate her own plans within her area.

Where a comprehensive plan already exists, there will be little difficulty, as the teachers will be actively interested in health teaching, using the health visitor and other members of the health team to deal with application in specific fields, such as child care, education for family life, human relationships or current medical problems. (Smoking and venereal disease are examples of two subjects needing specialist knowledge.)

If there is no overall policy, there are likely to be individual teachers who are enthusiastic, and every opportunity should be taken to work with them in making any plans. One health visitor working alone in two or three schools in her area, can only hope to reach a handful of school leavers, at the most, during the year, and some of the valuable occasions for teaching preventive measures (for example, concerning smoking) to the younger age groups will inevitably be lost. But working closely with teachers who are interested, the health visitor can extend her influence throughout the school for the appropriate age groups, utilizing her time more effectively by fitting into the curriculum where she is most needed. All children should be able to benefit from health education—boys as well as girls, and all age groups. This can only be done in close consultation with teachers, the health visitor making known the services available through the health department. Without this close liaison it is very easy for an enthusiastic health visitor, alive to the opportunities offered to her, to overload herself with teaching to the exclusion of other important visiting in the homes.

Thus the principles which should guide the health visitor when deciding upon her activities in the field of school health education are based upon the fact that she needs to make the most effective use of her time and skills in relation to the other priorities in the area and the needs of the school children. To carry out this policy she will need to make the most use of any scheme already in action, fitting into the team, or co-operating with the teachers, teaching where specialist knowledge is essential and offering her services in a consultative capacity.

If it appears that emphasis has been placed on her role as a health educator it is because this is the aspect of the work in the School Health Service which is growing and developing as the potential of the health visitor becomes more widely recognized; and as it becomes possible for some of her routine work to be delegated to assistants. (Some schools have actually appointed health visitors as full-time members of the teaching staff.)

As the accent of her work in the School Health Service has moved away from treatment, over the early years of the century, and the emphasis moved on to prevention rather than cure, it is now changing again, moving towards maintaining the early detection of defects and promoting good physical and mental health and the development of an integrated personality. If this aim is to be retained the health visitor will need to develop fully her role as a health educator in the School Health Service.

References

1. *The Health of the School Child*, 1958 and 1964, H.M.S.O.
2. Ministry of Health, Circular 12/65.
3. *Health Education,* Report, H.M.S.O., 1964.
4. *Health Education*, Ministry of Education (1958) Pamphlet 31, H.M.S.O.
5. *Health Education Journal*, volume 22, May 1964, and volume 22, November 1964.

Suggested Reading

Health Education, Education Pamphlet 31, H.M.S.O.
Childhood and Adolescence, A. J. HADFIELD (Pelican).
Journey Through Adolescence, DORIS ODLUM (Pelican).
Health In Education, Education Pamphlet 49, H.M.S.O.
Methods of Approach to School Children and Young People, G.M.OWEN, Midwife and
Health Visitor, Vol. 1, No. 8.

8. The Principles of Health Education

Grace Owen

The function of the health visitor was defined in the Jameson Report[1] as "health education and social advice". This means that she needs a full understanding of the principles of health education if she is to fulfil her function adequately, and also she needs to be able to apply them intelligently to all aspects of her work. It is only when general principles are fully appreciated that individuals are enabled to gain complete freedom from dogmatism in approach and to act on their own initiative as the situation demands. This flexible approach is essential in present-day health education.

Health education draws its empirical knowledge from a variety of disciplines, including medicine, physical sciences, psychology and sociology, and communicates this subject matter through the application of modern educational techniques.

In the words of the World Health Organization Expert Committee of 1954[2] it aims:

1. To make health a valued asset in the community.
2. To equip people with knowledge and skills that they can use to solve their health problems.
3. To promote the development of health services.

The ways in which people behave in relation to healthy living are influenced by a complex set of factors, as we shall see later, and therefore any approach to health education needs a knowledge of the situation, and rather special techniques to overcome resistances. The health visitor's whole approach to her work can be influenced by her concept of health education, thus it is important for her to understand its principles, and its broadest connotations and to appreciate her own role as a health educator.

We must first establish our definition of health education, so that we have our terms of reference clear. We may choose, simply, to define "health" as "wholeness", or to use the very apt definition to be found in the Ministry Pamphlet 31, on Health Education[3] which describes health as "a smooth functioning of body and mind, and a proper balance between the individual human being and his environment". This is a

74

realistic definition for our purposes as it allows a sense of achievement for those who are handicapped physically, or limited by their environment. "Education" is derived from the Latin *educo*, (or *e duco*) which suggests "leading" or "drawing out". Thus combining the two words we can define "health education" as a "process of leading individuals towards a state of health where they achieve a smooth functioning of body and mind and a proper balance between the individual human being and the environment". This gives us a precise description of our aim and also the sense of "leading" is in tune with present-day educational trends, doing away with any idea that dogmatic instruction is of value in health teaching, and emphasizing the need for the individual to respond, where necessary, by a change in behaviour.

In this chapter we shall look briefly at some historical and philosophical trends in the development of health education, which are helpful in understanding some of the factors influencing our current provisions. After discussing the opportunities available to the health visitor, we shall examine some educational principles and methods, and see how she can apply them in carrying out her function as a health educator.

Historical and Philosophical Trends

Man has been concerned with preventing disease and maintaining a healthy body for himself from the earliest days of history, and in the most primitive societies. We find evidence of this in many ancient historical records, sometimes the knowledge and experience of the physicians of the time exerting great influence, and at other times practice being associated with ritual, superstition, and religious customs. The same position can be seen today, to some extent, in the fact that in spite of our vast resources of scientific knowledge, medical evidence can be ignored in favour of beliefs influenced by custom and folklore, and these beliefs still dominate attitudes and behaviour in relation to health, even in civilized societies.

One of the earliest records of a code of health rules is to be found in the Mosaic writings of the Old Testament. Much of this Mosaic law, which later became Jewish ritual, was established for the maintenance of good community and personal health.

The Ancient civilizations of Greece and Rome had their codes for healthy living and much of their philosophy was modern, compared even with present day trends.

The Greeks believed in "education for wholeness" and Plato advocated teaching for expectant mothers and giving advice to young parents in the pre-natal clinic, suggesting expectant mothers should "take long walks". During the first 3 years of its life a child "must be happy, free from sorrow and pain as far as its childish desires permit ... taught by mild deprivations and the enjoyment of simple pleasures to find happiness in the middle way".[4]

Ancient Rome also had its traditions, and apart from the well-known association with heating, bathing and good plumbing in communal life, we find an emphasis on family life and the family as a unit, with great importance attached to the mother–child relationship. In no other civilization has maternal influence been so profound.[4]

The Hebrews, too, had a regard for the physical, mental and moral influences in the environment and the importance of stable family life.

These traditional ways of thinking became deeply embedded in the *mores* and customs of the people of these ancient civilizations, and much of their practice could be considered enlightened by present-day standards. This enlightenment, however, appeared to get lost in the obscurity of the Dark Ages and little is known about health education practice until the fifteenth and sixteenth centuries, when thinkers began to establish the importance of the relationship between behaviour and health and to compile rules for health. Salerno's eight doctrines of health were published over four centuries, and Galatio of Della Casa[5] established his rules for food care and handling, which could still be regarded as important today. The effects of disease and infection were, however, limited (apart from outbreaks of Plague) by the fact that people lived in scattered communities and communication was poor. The doctors of the eighteenth century knew little more than the physicians of the Ancient World.

But with industrialization came rapid changes, especially in Britain, where socio-economic and scientific advances, with increasing medical knowledge, were coupled with urbanization, overcrowding and insanitary conditions and the ravages of cholera and other diseases. During the nineteenth century increased medical knowledge made little impact because legislation was slow to take effect and the increased knowledge remained in the hands of the privileged few. With the increase of literacy in the early twentieth century came also a new awareness of the need for health education. There were attempts at teaching expectant mothers, and "hygiene" appeared on school timetables (often linked with teaching on temperance!). Florence Nightingale was among the first people to realize the value of teaching in the home, and with the growth of the health visiting profession new avenues here were pioneered and established.

The many improvements in physical health over the twentieth century are due to a combination of factors including the extension of social welfare provisions and education, and growth of scientific knowledge. Many of these social reforms have had an educational value in establishing new attitudes and beliefs, and changed patterns of behaviour leading to better health. Much of this success had been attributed to the patient teaching by all members of the Health and Social Services team, in the field of health education in this country, and parallel situations can be seen in other industrial societies.

We have already commented that the complex factors affecting health education demand a rather special approach. Firstly, we noticed that attitudes to health were often influenced by witchcraft, sorcery and superstition. This is understandable in primitive societies, but more surprising when we encounter superstitions in our own society, especially when we discover the strength these factors hold in some areas. An example is found in the widespread beliefs concerning harmful behaviour during menstruation and pregnancy in this country.

Often in other societies the beliefs held are even more illogical. One primitive tribe, for example, believes that eating oranges during pregnancy will harm the foetus. Their own health visitor was able to break down this fallacy eventually, when she married and herself became pregnant, and ate oranges constantly in public places, eventually producing a very healthy, normal baby! This was certainly an unusual method, but serves to illustrate the point in question.

As already noted, various religions have formulated codes of behaviour for health, some of which have been ritualized and assimilated into the culture of the society, surviving long after new discoveries have rendered them obsolete. Where such beliefs exist and are contrary to present-day knowledge, they must be respected and new ways of overcoming the difficulties have to be sought. Many of these beliefs are associated with diet and food handling.

The effects of custom, tradition and culture often give rise to deep-seated prejudices and attitudes which must be understood before they can be broken down and re-established. This is often very apparent in patterns of childrearing and socialization, and examples can be found in a number of recent surveys, notably that of John and Elizabeth Newsom in *Patterns of Infant Care* in Nottingham.[6]

Now, in addition to improved knowledge in medicine and environmental health, we have more understanding of sociological and psychological problems involved in health education, and also know better how to approach them from an educational point of view. Early this century the need was for wide dissemination of elementary facts about health and hygiene and methods used concentrated on this, often in a dogmatic way. Today, it is realized a new approach is needed. Most people are literate, and have access to factual knowledge and many know basic principles, but do not apply them, but those who do not know, may be apathetic or unaware of their need, and therefore resistant. Therefore the challenge is different from that of the past. We still need to inform, of course, where necessary, but generally speaking we must go further and seek to encourage people to act on the information given[7] and this involves knowing the techniques of changing attitudes and faulty beliefs.

It must be remembered that in applying these techniques we may be exposed to criticism from those who feel this is something akin to the subtleties employed in advertising, therefore the health educator must utilize only the facts, as they are known at the time, presenting them in their entirety and without bias. Health education should not be an opportunity for the unscrupulous person to sell his own ideas and opinions.

Health Education in Britain Today

The statutory provision for health education in Britain is found mainly in the 1936 Public Health Act (sect. 179) and the 1946 National Health Service Act (sect. 21–28). These acts do not define the position clearly, but it is implied in the phraseology that the services provided will certainly necessitate health education and local authorities are given power to carry this out.

The Central Council of Health Education is a national co-ordinating body which assists local authorities, by offering in-service training, literature, and equipment, and provides facilities for research. Most health education is carried on by the staff of local health authorities, health visitors, medical officers of health, and nurses, assisted by teachers, parents and others. Many authorities now have health education departments, with a qualified health education officer in charge and responsible to the medical officer of health for co-ordination and practice in the area, assessing the needs, planning campaigns, providing equipment, staff and training, and evaluating results. At international level health education is carried out by World Health Organization, officers being appointed at regional level to organize field work. Before development can be effective it is essential to assess local need, customs and belief; and to educate the people to accept new ideas, which can otherwise be useless. There are three main channels for health education; the individual, the group and the community.

Health Education for the Individual

The individual situation usually arises in the face-to-face consultation. Much of the health visitor's work in the health education field falls into this category, as she is constantly giving guidance in the fields of child care and development, family relationships and preventive medicine, so laying the foundations for positive physical and mental health.

The principles of interviewing, discussed elsewhere in this book, are directly applicable to this situation and inseparable from any techniques used. Individual health education has one major advantage, in the fact that if often arises as a direct response to an expression of individual need, or it can be directly related to the interests of the person concerned, and in this way learning is likely to be facilitated. This can, of course, be outweighed if the wrong approach is made and the recipient feels a sense of criticism is implied. Difficulties arise when the situation presented is so complex, that the health visitor does not know which problem to deal with first. She will do well to select the most urgent needs and deal only with them and return at a later date for the rest, or there will be resentment or apathy, if too much is tackled. In all individual education the principles discussed later in this chapter will be found useful.

Group Health Education

This affords a wide scope for the health visitor and is an interesting and rewarding aspect of her work. She may find she has access to groups already existing in the community, or alternatively opportunities arise to create new groups. Existing groups will include those in the personal health and social services, such as expectant mothers, school children or parent–teacher's associations. Various societies and organizations, such as the Red Cross and St. Johns, Women's Institutes, church groups or youth clubs, may often welcome the health visitor's assistance from time to time.

The family is more than ever regarded as an important unit for health education today, especially the mother as she is concerned with all the basic issues of living, such as food, health, and child-rearing, and her attitude may well influence the family as a whole.

It is often argued that group health education is time-consuming owing to the need for preparation, but against this, we must set the economies offered. One can reach ten or fifteen people in a group in the same time as one person alone, and sometimes more effectively, because of the cumulative value of group interaction between members themselves. Also group decisions tend to be stronger, and are known to extend beyond the limits of the initial group involved. An example of this was seen recently in a village mothers' club, where a group decision was made concerning children's footwear. The effects of this decision were strong enough to persuade many others attending the clinic, and to influence the local shoe store in the type of footwear offered for sale.

Groups also have a therapeutic potential for those who belong. Shy people find friends and nervous ones gain reassurance when finding their anxieties are common to all. Tensions are released and opportunities provided for self-expression and learning through activity. There is also the fact that members learn much from each other if discussion is skilfully encouraged and directed.

Such groups are an asset to the work of any health visitor, providing as they do a basic unit for health education, and also the advantage of getting to know many people on her area better. This encourages them to approach her with confidence when needing help, and the barriers have already been dispensed with, which again can reduce time spent on visits. If she takes advantage of invitations to existing groups her acceptance in the community will be widened, as her potential is realized. Most health visitors will find themselves at some time, teaching a group of expectant mothers. Such groups may be organized by a local authority, hospital or clinic, and the health visitor and midwife may share the responsibility. Usually, some form of relaxation and exercise for childbirth, or psycho-prophylaxis is offered, accompanied by a series of discussions on pregnancy, labour, and management of the new baby.

Difficulty may be experienced in getting the mothers to attend early enough in pregnancy to make the teaching worthwhile, but in some areas it has been possible to overcome this with the co-operation of industrial firms and employers, who are prepared to allow time off for the expectant mother. Fathers, now, are very often included in evening groups.

The programme needs to be flexible and adapted to the needs of the group, according to their social background and intelligence. In certain areas elementary information on preparation of the layette may be essential but in other areas this can be dispensed with and other topics given priority. Basic teaching on health in pregnancy, normal labour, feeding and the application of relaxation techniques are essential for most groups, however.

Appropriate teaching aids, such as the *Birth Atlas*, films and filmstrips are helpful, but generally discussion is easily stimulated as members of the group have a strong common interest and are eager to learn.

Recent research carried out by the Royal College of Midwives[8] gives evidence of the needs of mothers, and the current situation, essential information to any health visitor interested in these groups.

Mothers' clubs or parents' groups may be an excellent starting point for health education for the health visitor. She may find a group already flourishing when she goes into a new area, or may be able to establish one if the need is apparent. It may be helpful to have an idea how to create such a group, as much of its success depends upon the way it is established.

It will first be necessary to assess the need of the area, the interests and the wishes of prospective members, and then an informal meeting can be arranged with a few keen mothers to discuss proposals. The availability of accommodation must be investigated if no suitable clinic premises are available, which means funds will be needed, and methods of financial support must be discussed. In many areas there are schemes sponsored by the local authority, which enable the groups to join an association and gain financial support, or direct grants may be available. Funds can be raised by annual subscriptions and small weekly contributions to cover current expenditure.

Groups may meet in the afternoons, when a crèche is essential for toddlers, but these groups are not easy to run from an educational point of view and many clubs prefer evening meetings. Mothers are often distracted, or anxious to get away afternoons, but evenings they can leave the family behind and tiredness soon disappears as they relax and get absorbed in their activity.

Frequency of meetings varies, some meeting monthly, fortnightly, or weekly—the latter often providing for quicker integration and better continuity.

An elected committee is essential, composed of a chairman who is able to meet and introduce speakers and act as general leader, a treasurer to deal with finance, and a secretary, who should be able to compose an acceptable letter and keep accurate minutes. Other officers can be appointed to suit local desires, but the health visitor should establish that she is an ex-officio member at all committees and the annual general meeting.

A constitution is important if only to regularize procedure, limit membership, and safeguard the type of activity desired. A good balance is achieved with 75 per cent health education and 25 per cent social activity. A group so established will soon function well and is self-supporting in the absence of the health visitor, who will find she can often act in an advisory capacity, helping on some occasions with teaching, but finding the routine work ably dealt with by group members. Several groups can be covered this way, whereas if the health visitor is too involved with administration she will find it limits her usefulness in wider spheres.

Programmes can include lectures, discussions, panels or brains trusts, and films or demonstrations are often welcome. A wide range of topics is popular, including all aspects of child care and development, family relationships and care of the aged or handicapped. Attitudes to mental health and use of the social services are good discussion topics and many professional people and commercial firms make their services available to such groups.

A health visitor who has a group of this kind will find her initial hard work amply rewarded as the group becomes self-supporting and a focus for activity in relation to health teaching.

Sometimes there are opportunities for youth club work. This demands rather special skills from the health educator, but some health visitors find scope here for their talent. The members of the group vary widely in tastes and intelligence but most young people are needing some sort of guidance in adjusting to standards at work, differing from those at school. They have, comparatively speaking, plenty to spend and little responsibility. They may have inquiring minds and be ready to discuss topics that interest them, but are often ill-informed and vulnerable in relation to health and moral problems, such as venereal disease[9] and drug addiction.

The field is wide open and challenging for the health visitor who is invited to enter this type of group work. The important thing is that she should have a liking for young people and be able to accept them just as she finds them, and be prepared to answer their questions frankly. She may be able to guide their choice of programme, and introduce the use of special techniques such as role play, remembering above all the importance of a permissive atmosphere. Many members of these groups will themselves be parents in the next few years, and thus it is an important group for the health educator.

We have already discussed elsewhere the principles of school health education for the health visitor, and it is sufficient here just to remind ourselves that school children are the only truly "captive" audience we have, and once the child leaves school our chances of getting him to join other groups for health education purposes are rather remote, and only comparatively small numbers of the population are reached.

These are the most frequently existing groups to which the health visitor has access, but she may well be asked to assist with other associations, such as Old People's Clubs, Red Cross Cadets or Guides, either giving a series of talks or helping with plans for health education.

The Community

The health visitor will be concerned inevitably with health education in the community, sometimes participating actively but in any case needing to appreciate current activities and trends. She may actually be involved in health campaigns at a local or national level, either in helping with displays or demonstrations, lecturing, or assisting in planning and exhibition work. There are often specific age groups to be reached through a special effort, where they are not available in any of the groups previously described. An example of this could be a road safety campaign, particularly aimed at the young motor cyclist, or a health campaign designed for those in their middle years. The latter is a particularly difficult group to reach any other way, most of them being busy career people or disinterested in group activity, but the *Cohen Report*[7] draws attention to their vulnerability and need for health education.

The health visitor needs to keep well informed on current literature, and in touch with modern methods and techniques of communication, and to have some idea of what goes on on radio, television and in magazines. While broadcast material reaches a very wide audience, its educational value is somewhat limited and can be improved by reinforcement in individual and group situations, where discussion is possible.

Principles of Communication — Methods, Techniques and Preparation

From the beginning of her training, the student health visitor will be gaining factual information to equip her for her future function, but this alone is not sufficient. She must understand the principles of communicating this information in such a way that response is achieved, where necessary, resulting in changed behaviour patterns. The *Cohen Report on Health Education*[7] (which can be studied by every student with advantage) states that we must do more than provide information—"we must seek to influence people to act on the advice and information given, and further, to counter measures injurious to health". It stresses the need for understanding and application of appropriate techniques, and with this end in view, the health visitor will need to know factors governing the learning processes and suitable educational principles and to apply them to the situations she finds.

While not attempting here to discuss educational psychology, we may do well to remind ourselves briefly of some principles essential to the health visitor's work in health education. Learning is a change of behaviour occurring as a result of past experiences and brought about by interaction between the individual and the environment, thus indicating the importance of response in the learning situation.

Many factors influence the learning processes and motivation is one of the most apparent ones. People learn readily what they want to learn and when they want to learn and thus are motivated by interest in themselves and the basic needs of their bodies. We have an illustration of this in the expectant mother who is strongly motivated to learn all she can about her baby's arrival because it matters to her intensely, to know what is happening to her body. The biological needs for survival, self-preservation and avoidance of pain are strong ones, and physical discomfort such as cold, hunger or fatigue can have an inhibiting effect on learning. The need for security is also a strong motivating factor, and this is why anything that increases confidence and dispels fear is likely to aid learning. The need for acceptance and respect, too, are concerned and we notice this in the mothers who are eager to learn how to be successful with problems such as toilet training or temper tantrums, where success carries a high status value.

Sometimes if motivation is weak the teacher can strengthen it by introducing new goals or aims with some knowledge of achievement or a competitive element, and these are especially helpful when dealing with children.

Where any of these interests are strong they help to secure and retain attention. When we are deeply absorbed in something that is worthwhile to us, our attention is held to the exclusion of distractions. It may be quite easy for the teacher to hold interest if the group members want to learn, but much more difficult with a captive audience. Therefore we need to know how to arouse and maintain interest.

Attention is quite an important factor in learning as we learn most readily the things we attend to most thoroughly, and we tend to select from our environment and pay attention to things that matter to us. Certain stimuli, such as unusual or changing ones (for example, movement or colour) are known to attract attention and we can apply this when we especially need to arouse interest, or in the use of visual aids.

Attention and perception are closely linked—we perceive more readily the things we want to see, and our willingness to acquire new ideas is governed by things we have previously learned, therefore pleasant or unpleasant experiences are important. Thus the mother who has experienced a difficult delivery will need a lot of help in gaining a positive approach to a second pregnancy. We perceive and attend more readily to things which we recognize, and therefore it is helpful to follow the simple rule of moving from the known to the unknown in teaching. This also assists understanding and insight—two more important factors.

The fact that difficulty is experienced when a person is faced with something he does not wish to learn (unconsciously or consciously) is of importance to the health visitor, who is constantly dealing with subjects about which individuals may have deep-seated prejudices, attitudes, or fears.

The importance of activity in learning is especially relevant with younger children who cannot concentrate for long periods and when there is likely to be any difficulty in maintaining interest. It also assists people to become absorbed and involved in the task, and to learn by experience, or trial and error, the best way of doing things for themselves. Action also helps to reinforce a concept that has just been learned and activity provides a knowledge of progress and a chance to correct errors. It is especially useful when it comes to practising skills where constant repetition is needed. All this can be applied to many situations, for example, when a health visitor shows a mother how to prepare a baby's feed correctly; and then encourages her as she tries out the procedure for herself. The most effective type of group activity is that which demands a personal response from each individual member.

There are also individual differences between learners which can affect progress and these include some factors already mentioned, such as motivation and past experience, and others such as intelligence and motivation.

This brief outline offers some basic principles for the health visitor's application in any educational situation, and they will need to be considered in any preparation of material.

Methods, Techniques and Teaching Aids

Again, this section should not be regarded as an exhaustive exposition on teaching principles, but simply a guide to some useful methods of approach for the health visitor.

Selection of method will be made according to the aim or purpose in view, the type of group and subject. Much depends upon whether the intention is to communicate facts or to attempt to influence attitudes and behaviour. It can be a combination of these two but is more often the latter in health education. It is difficult to communicate factual knowledge to an apathetic or unconcerned audience, and often more effective to apply the principles we have discussed, arousing interest and encouraging an active role in learning and discussion. A dogmatic approach could build up further resistance.

Hence the formal lecture is rarely used in health education except perhaps to students or professional people who are highly motivated to learn, even so discussion is often combined with a lecture.

Short talks may be given, but it is now widely recognized (see, again, the *Cohen Report*[7]) that the Socratic method of discussion and question should be used in addition.

Group discussion is now the most popular and effective method available. It offers opportunities for exchanging ideas, changing faulty attitudes and correcting misconceptions. It provides a channel for self-expression, and gaining insight into solving problems, with the advantage of more effective decision, and is especially useful in handling highly controversial subjects. Adequate preparation, however, is essential so that the leader can be equipped with necessary information, and is prepared to be flexible in approach.

Variations on discussion include the "brains trust" or "panel" type of discussion. In the former, a group of experts face the audience and spontaneous discussion of questions presented takes place. More thought and preparation goes into the "panel" discussion, which is skilfully guided by the chairman and allows for audience participation. The "buzz group" technique is useful for breaking up a large group and encouraging participation. Often these are formed spontaneously from four to six members sitting nearest each other, being given a topic to discuss for a few moments only. Sometimes a member of the small group is asked to share findings with the larger group, or the teacher may, by use of questions, bring out the points he wishes to discuss. Its main value lies in allowing participation and stimulating active discussion, or alleviating a situation in a large group where boredom is apparent or response poor.

Role-playing is a technique rapidly gaining popularity, especially as it is widely used in schools. It is accepted as a very effective method of teaching where human relationships are concerned, as it provides opportunities to act out situations that may well occur in real life. It has the advantage that participants can either "be themselves" or take on the role of another, and experiment with a new situation, self-consciousness being minimized. The whole session needs careful thought and planning by the leader, to ensure success, but the actual role-playing is spontaneous. The leader can prepare the situation for discussion, or it may arise in the course of a lesson. Usually participants are given a few seconds to decide upon allocation of roles, and then proceed to act out the situation. The leader may stop them after 2 or 3 minutes or as soon as a few valuable foci for discussion have emerged. Sometimes a second group can give a different interpretation, and then the whole group can assess it, discussing the various implications. This method is particularly suited to young people, children, groups dealing with human relationships, or attitudes to authority, and helps in resolving individual problems.

Teaching aids may be used in conjunction with any of the methods already described, but it must always be remembered that they are only "aids" to teaching and must be supported by the appropriate approach.

In areas where a health education department exists the health visitor has access to expert advice on the production and use of teaching aids, also the services of artists and technicians, and necessary equipment. She will need herself to understand the principles of using these aids, selecting those suitable for the type of audience and relevant to the subject matter. They should also be topical, attractive and colourful and clearly visible and above all, efficiently produced, as they inevitably have to compete with the commercial art of today, if health is to be "sold" as a valuable commodity.

Films, filmstrips, slides and tape-recordings can all be used if properly introduced and supported by discussion. Flannelgraphs, plastographs and models can be usefully incorporated in short talks especially for children. Puppets are also popular, allowing children to participate in preparation and script writing. Groups of adults will often join in a project, producing their own films or slides or preparing a demonstration for exhibition use.

The personality of the teacher herself is an important aid to teaching, especially as individual skills are developed. The proper and natural use of voice and gesture, and an attractive appearance are assets to any teacher, and a lively, friendly personality goes a long way to creating a relaxed atmosphere in the classroom.

The apt use of question and illustration should not be forgotten when preparing notes. It is difficult to frame questions spontaneously and they will aid discussion more effectively if one first decides whether they should be provocative, or open-ended, and ensures that they do not presuppose a certain answer.

Preparation of Material

Whatever methods, techniques or aids are selected, good preparation is essential to achieve success. It helps to give confidence and makes for efficient use of time and sequence of thought and ideas. It ensures accuracy, and proper use of aids, and provides a framework within which a skilled teacher can then afford to be flexible according to the needs of the group, and still achieve the aim in view.

Principles of good preparation involve careful consideration of the group, the subject and the relevant educational techniques and principles. It is a good idea to take three large sheets of paper and assemble rough notes on these three points before making a final copy. We need to know several things about the group, including their sex, average age and intelligence, social and cultural background and previous knowledge. The group is the most important element in the teaching situation. Next we need to consider the type of subject — whether factual or emotive, and to decide our aims in dealing with it. Factual material will be collected and selected, seeking for a logical sequence of main ideas. We need to consider relevant educational principles in order to decide upon a method and aids. For example, if we have a large group of school children below average intelligence, we need to remember that they will learn best if interested, and actively involved, as their motivation may be weak. Therefore we select an approach most likely to arouse and maintain interest, we try to "make it matter" to them, and use such methods as buzz groups, or projects to ensure participation.

Always we can apply the three basic rules, planning our material to proceed from the known to the unknown, simple to complex, and whole to parts.

This approach ensures intelligent application of principles and we can then assemble our notes. Various methods are used but basically all plan for an introduction, development and summary or conclusion. The relevant information concerning the group, aims and aids used, can be selected and included in the title page, which is useful if notes are to be kept for future reference.

It is easier to write notes on one side of the paper only, numbering pages and pinning firmly together. Good spacing is essential, main and subheadings being clearly numbered and underlined, with all factual material in note formation. A wide column can be left down one side of the page, to include the aids used, such as questions or visual aids, at the appropriate point in the text. Other notes such as references, or diagrams may be added at the discretion of the teacher, or some indication given of any material which is essential, or that which can be omitted if time is short.

It should always be remembered that notes are simply a framework within which the teacher may be as flexible as the needs and response of the group demand. Good preparation should have ensured that the teacher is familiar with his material and knows what he wants to say, and what he aims to do.

When actually talking or leading discussion the introduction is important, as this is when good contact is established with the group, and members are likely to decide whether or not the next half hour is going to be worthwhile to them, and worth their attention. Reading material, or learning subject matter by heart is not the best approach for a health educator, and most health visitors will find that experience and maturity make it relatively easy to talk spontaneously from well-prepared notes once *rapport* is established. It helps to look at all members of the group to gain contact and confidence and all this gives the leader an awareness of group reactions, allowing for adjustment, and change of techniques. Nervousness, inevitable for beginners, can be controlled by relaxed breathing and concentration on the needs of the group.

Special techniques are helpful in group discussion, the group always being informally arranged, the leader being seated as one of the group. The leader's functions include introducing the subject and ensuring that the necessary ground is covered and steering the group from one point to another at the appropriate time. Faulty statements will need correction and points clarified, and a permissive atmosphere should be created so that all members feel free to express their ideas. It is as opinions are expressed that individuals are able to discover any inadequacies and realize the need for further information to remedy a faulty approach. An awareness of need then makes the subject matter especially relevant. Weaker members may need encouragement, and talkative ones will need skilful handling. When the subject is a controversial one the leader will do well to avoid stating opinions at first, and will by use of questions and guidance of discussion, encourage an exchange of views, and search for new knowledge. In this way, as additional information becomes available, a group decision may well emerge, establishing a new course of action.

Individuals may gain insight into their own problems and attitudes will be changed, and this will probably give rise to healthy argument and some apparent resentment at times. The introduction of fresh information at the point where attitudes are breaking down, will assist in establishing new ones which will need reinforcement by the leader, whose function is to remain at all times unobtrusively in control of the situation.

Many health visitors find group discussion the most valuable technique for the type of work they are engaged in, and develop their own skills and potential in leading groups of all kinds and find this a stimulating and rewarding field.

Assessment and Evaluation

Discussion on the principles of health education would be incomplete without some reference to the usefulness of evaluation. Time and energy have often been wasted in the past by teaching sporadically according to the interests of the health visitor.

There are two aspects involved here—first of all we need to assess the needs of the community or group. This can be done by a general survey of the area using the tools of modern sociology, or by investigating statistics at the local health department. Secondly, we can attempt to evaluate the results of our efforts, assessing the knowledge and attitudes of people before and again after a health education campaign. This kind of evaluation is not easy to obtain accurately, but attempts have been made in Aberdeen (1960),[10] and also by Jeffreys and Westaway (1960–61)[11] on smoking habits among school children.

In the absence of any empirical survey of this kind the health visitor can attempt to assess her priorities in the light of her knowledge of her area. Local statistics will reveal current problems needing attention and she can concentrate her efforts on these topics, and on the section of the community where the need is greatest. Evaluation is difficult, but over a period of time, statistics may indicate she has made progress.

With individual groups it is easier to discover their needs and interests and assess the situation after teaching, by means of a questionnaire. Evaluation is a useful tool and intelligently applied can ensure that priorities are dealt with in home, school, or community.

It is not necessary here to engage in detailed discussion on the subject matter involved in current topics for health education, especially as this is constantly changing and adequate information can be gained elsewhere, some reading being suggested at the end of this chapter.

In examining these general principles of health education, it is evident that they apply to all aspects of health visiting, and every health visitor is in some way involved. To a few, health education is unattractive and time-consuming, but to most, it is an extremely interesting and challenging sphere of work. The application of these principles will ensure that the health visitor utilizes every available opportunity, creating new ones as and when they are needed, and does this, keeping a true sense of perspective concerning her priorities in all aspects of her work.

References

1. *An Enquiry into Health Visiting*, H.M.S.O., 1956.
2. Expert Committee on Health Education of the Public (1954). World Health Organization, Technical Report Series No. 89.
3. *Health Education*, Ministry of Education (1958), Pamphlet 31, H.M.S.O.
4. *Ancient Education and Today*, E. B. CASTLE (Pelican).
5. *A Textbook of Health Education*, DENIS PIRRIE and A. J. DALZELL-WARD.
6. *Patterns of Infant Care*, JOHN and ELIZABETH NEWSOM (Pelican).
7. *Health Education Report*, H.M.S.O., 1964.
8. *Preparation for Parenthood*, Royal College of Midwives.
9. *The Sexual Behaviour of Young People*, MICHAEL SCHOFIELD.
10. *Evaluation of a Scheme of Health Education*, I. A. Q. MacQueen, Medical Officer 103, 295.
11. "Catch them before they start", M. JEFFREYS and W. R. WESTAWAY (1961), *Health Education Journal,* Vol. 19. No. 1.

Suggested Reading

A Textbook of Health Education, DENIS PIRRIE and A. J. DALZELL-WARD.
Common Sense About Smoking, FLETCHER/COLE/JEGER/WOOD (Penguin Special).
Cancer, R. J. G. HARRIS.
Venereal Diseases, R. S. MORTON (Pelican).
Discrimination and Popular Culture, DENYS THOMPSON (Pelican).
The Psychology of Learning, R. BORGER and A. E. M. SEABORNE (Pelican).
Alcoholism, RESSEL and WALTON (Pelican).

Appendix I. Training Notes

AT THE time of writing this book, the following are the conditions of entry for health visitor training:
1. State registered nurse.
2. State certified midwife or Part I of the Central Midwives Board examination or a recognized obstetric training, together with a minimum of five O-levels in the General Certificate of Education or its equivalent.

The duration of training is one calendar year. This consists of one academic year, followed by 3 months supervised practice. During the academic year one-third of the time is spent in practical work. Registration will be granted to successful candidates on the recommendation of the training unit, following a satisfactory report on the supervised practice.

The examination consists of written papers covering the syllabus and an oral examination in which there is discussion and the presentation of family case studies and a project or a day book.

Appendix II. Syllabus for the Training of Health Visitors

THE syllabus laid down by the Council for the Training of Health Visitors as follows.

Section I   Development of the Individual

In broad terms the changes associated with the life cycle and the disorders and problems commonly met with in health visiting practice.
Elementary genetics.
The norms of intellectual, emotional and physical development of the young child and in the school years.
Physical and emotional aspects of periods of change, e.g. puberty and middle life.
The mature personality.
Effects of ageing on general capacity, the special senses and intellectual processes.
Methods of estimating and measuring individual capacities at varying ages.

Section II   The Individual in the Group

An introduction to the study of society.
The family as a social institution.
Its functions and relationships with other institutions.
Regional and class differences.
Activities and power structure within the family.

Section III   Development of Social Policy

Poverty in the nineteenth century, public attitudes to its causes and relief.
The introduction of social insurance.
The growth of the health services —
    a. The hospital system, including provision for the mentally disordered;
    b. Environmental services and local government responsibilities;

c. Services for mothers and young children;
d. Services for the handicapped and aged in the community.

Education and the service of youth.
The care of the deprived child, child life protection and control of adoption.
The role of voluntary organizations.

Section IV   Social Aspects of Health and Disease

An introduction to demography and to epidemiology of infectious and non-infectious disease, the uses of statistics, surveys.
The personal and environmental health services.
Current medical problems and their implications for the community services.
International health.

Section V   Principles and Practice of Health Visiting

The Role of the Health Visitor in Contemporary Society
Her spheres of work, their extent and limitations with regard to the family in general. Her role in the maternity and child welfare and school services, with particular reference to the promotion of mental health, the control of infectious disease, the elderly, and in general medical practice.

The Objectives in Health Visiting
The assessments of the health prospects for the individual, treatment, care and the amelioration of adverse factors in the environment, or the introduction of other services to achieve this.

Health Visiting
Assessment of priorities in visiting.
Establishing a relationship with the family.
The use of the interview.
Techniques and methods used in various types of interview in home and clinic.
Relationship with workers in allied services based on a knowledge of their functions and sphere of work, means of communication and techniques of referral.
Preparation of reports, case conferences, record keeping.
Responsibilities in clinic and school, including day-to-day administration of the former, integration and co-operation in general medical practice.
Relationship to auxiliary workers with the local health authority and local welfare authority services.

Health Education

Present-day aims and scope of health education and the health visitor's contribution to this.

Elementary principles of educational psychology and their application to individual and group teaching at various ages.

Methods of teaching, including group techniques for the amelioration of individual and family problems.

Index